WHO TAKES PROZAC?

You'd be amazed. Since its introduction, over 11 million patients worldwide and 5 million in the United States have taken Prozac. These people range from children to adolescents to the elderly—from lifelong depressives who, with the help of Prozac, are beginning for the first time to structure their lives in responsible ways, to many highly successful, productive people who have had from one to numerous depressions in their lifetime.

Name any randomly chosen group of successful people in society, business, politics, or the arts, and it is likely that 20 percent to 30 percent are either taking or have taken Prozac at some point over the last several years. People of all classes, races, and religions have benefited and talked about the miraculous effects of Prozac in reversing their despair, chronic lack of pleasure, poor functioning, and persistent low level depression.

No matter where you live in the United States, you probably know someone who has taken it ... or should be considering it.

PROZAC

DR. RONALD R. FIEVE, M.D.

AVON BOOKS ◆ NEW YORK

To my daughters, Lara and Vanessa, and to my patients

PROZAC is an original publication of Avon Books. This work has never before appeared in book form.

The ideas, procedures, and suggestions in this book are intended to supplement, not replace, the medical advice of a trained medical professional. All matters regarding your health require medical supervision. Consult your physician before adopting the suggestions in this book, as well as any condition that may require diagnosis or medical attention. The author and publisher disclaim any liability arising directly or indirectly from the use of this book.

AVON BOOKS
A division of
The Hearst Corporation
1350 Avenue of the Americas
New York, New York 10019

Copyright © 1994 by Dr. Ronald Fieve
Published by arrangement with the author
Library of Congress Catalog Card Number: 93-94072
ISBN: 0-380-77718-5

First Avon Books Printing: April 1994

AVON TRADEMARK REG. U.S. PAT. OFF. AND IN OTHER COUNTRIES, MARCA REGISTRADA, HECHO EN U.S.A.

Printed in the U.S.A.

RA 10 9 8 7 6 5 4 3 2 1

Acknowledgments

I would like to give special thanks and appreciation to Nancy Hathaway for her superior work, cheerful attitude, and tireless energy in working with me all hours of the night and day in order to complete this manuscript. Many, many thanks.

I would also like to acknowledge my wonderful, conscientious, and loyal staff, which is responsible for running and coordinating three offices in New York City. In particular, I am grateful to Motria Milanytch, my personal research secretary and administrative assistant at the New York State Psychiatric Institute; Nancy Rao, my private practice nurse at the Atchley Pavilion, Columbia Presbyterian Medical Center; my private practice nurse, Bernadette Mannion, and my practice administrator, Lara Fieve, both at the Foundation for Depression and Manic Depression; Lori Thievon, director of business development for Fieve Clinical Services, which has participated for over two decades in the development of new antidepressant agents; Annamarie Schlegel and Maura del Bene, my drug study research nurses; Audrey Benjamin, Edna Spoor, and my nurse administrator Cynthia Craft;

Drs. Eric Peselow, Edward Berklehammer, Patrick Murphy, Chris Reiss, Edie Solomon, and, especially, Deborah Deliyannides for her work with my patients. I would also like to thank Lawrence Hughes, publisher of *Moodswing* and my editorial consultant for this book; Bob Mecoy, my editor at Avon Books; and my wife, Katia.

Contents

Preface

I made the decision to write this book some eight years after I began researching the use of Prozac in clinical depression. In 1985, I had agreed to enroll 120 depressed patients in a Prozac study and to be one of ten independent investigators across the country who would strictly follow a research protocol. The purpose was to see if Prozac was indeed effective in depression and to compare it to the standard antidepressant drug Tofranil (generically known as imipramine) and to placebo. Furthermore, side effects were to be strictly monitored and reported to a human rights committee as well as to Eli Lilly, the sponsor of the study.

This was a particularly exciting research study for me to participate in, because previously I had spent my academic career at Columbia Presbyterian Medical Center in New York City investigating the use of lithium carbonate, a mood stabilizer for depression and manic depression, as well as other antidepressants. Prozac represented the first of a new class of antidepressant compounds called selective serotonin reuptake inhibitors (SSRIs). I wanted to be in on the ground floor of its investigation, since I knew that the older drugs I'd used for many years produced a number of very unpleasant side effects including dry mouth, constipation, blurred vision, dizziness, sexual problems, and, most important to patients, weight gain. Prozac, according to everything I had read in the scientific literature in the early 1980s, had a milder side effect profile. In addition, some patients not only didn't gain weight with Prozac, they lost it.

Several years later, an analysis of the pooled data from the original study showed Prozac to be as effective as the standard antidepressant imipramine which I and thousands of other psychiatrists had used for over thirty years. Both Prozac and imipramine worked better than placebo, and, as had been predicted, the Prozac patients experienced a startling absence of side effects compared to the imipramine patients. This immediately made me think that Prozac would be the preferred drug of choice for depressed patients of the future.

A few years later, after Prozac had been marketed and I had begun to prescribe it for the depressed patients in my private practice, I started to get a feel for Prozac's distinct advantages and disadvantages. From a therapeutic point of view, I found Prozac to be as effective as the standard antidepressant drugs that had been used since 1958 by most psychiatrists. Moreover, after comparing Prozac to the older compounds, I found it was nontoxic to the heart and required only one capsule a day for most people instead of three to six. In addition, overdosing on Prozac to the point of death was almost impossible. Most important to the average clinically depressed patient, it produced minimal side effects. Furthermore, many patients lost weight on Prozac.

By early 1994, I had used Prozac on over three hundred patients and observed four distinct groups within that population:

- As with other antidepressant compounds, 30% to 35% of the patients on Prozac were nonresponsive and often needed to be switched to one of the older classic antidepressant drugs.

- As with other drugs, a small percentage of Prozac patients in the above group complained of side effects and on their own discontinued the drug before the next visit.

- From a therapeutic standpoint, a group of clinically depressed persons emerged who were Prozac responders. After one to six weeks' treatment on Prozac (typically two to four weeks), I found that their depressed symptoms were relieved. These patients reported feeling their normal selves, leading to a renewal of their usual work and personal relationships.

- Finally, and of particular interest to me, a small group of patients reported an almost immediate lifting of the depression followed by a sense of brightening and a feeling of extraordinary well-being. I call them antidepressant hyperresponders. For the people in this latter group, Prozac appears to offer nothing less than transformation.

Prozac offers great promise and raises many questions. This book provides the answers to the questions most frequently asked by patients, their families, and physicians.

• 1 •

Transformation, Restoration, and the Psychopharmacological Miracle of Our Time

In my private practice, I have seen a few patients utterly changed by Prozac, lifted from the deepest despair into an even-tempered, confident optimism. Their lives improved so suddenly and dramatically that they *seemed* to have new personalities. More often, however, the changes are less spectacular. The patient returns from the paralysis of depression to a normal level of functioning. It is a shift back to wellness, a restoration of the self rather than a transformation.

One of my patients, K.S., is a 36-year-old former singer who had struggled for many years with "an undertow of depression." Born in the Midwest, she was sent to boarding school between the ages of 12 and 18, during which time her mother divorced, remarried, and moved to the East Coast with her new husband. After an Ivy League college education, K.S. sang in the chorus of a Broadway show, performed on television, and by age 26 went on a national tour. But ultimately, depression began to pull her down. "I was sent to see one doctor after another because I was supposed to be very nervous; finally one psychiatrist gave me mild tranquilizers, which didn't help, and then Thorazine," she recalled. "Later I found out that Thorazine is a drug that should be given only to psychotic patients and schizophrenics. Instead, I should have been given an antidepressant. With Thorazine I couldn't sing. I stopped taking it because it changed my facial expression, made my arms and legs stiff, and I even put on ten pounds. Needless to say, I also stopped seeing the doctor."

For the next two years, K.S. remained down, functioning poorly. "Then I became increasingly disturbed, terribly unhappy, which must have been a deepening of the same old depression."

She underwent treatment with several psychiatrists who gave her antidepressant medications that did not work. In addition, she saw two different psychologists for psychotherapy. Throughout the medication and psychotherapy treatments, K.S. stated, "I was never happy, although after spending close to $10,000, I did gain a few insights. Whenever anything nice would happen to me, I would wonder why the depression did not go away. It was as if I had a dark cloud hanging over me and the treatment never touched it. I just couldn't function."

K.S.'s history revealed high energy as well as sustained periods of achievement during her teens and early twenties. Her family history included an uncle who had been treated for manic depression and a cousin who had committed suicide. With these two latter clues in mind, my experience allowed me to predict that K.S. would probably benefit from small doses of Prozac. This prediction was based on the fact that she had not only a diagnosis of chronic depression but also a past history of energetic, outgoing moods (hyperthymia) and a family history of manic depression.

The change came swiftly. "Within a week I started to feel much better," K.S. reported. "I decided I would try to swim. I decided that I really didn't want to die. I wanted to go on living. I decided to use the energy I had in the morning to start cooking again, since I had once been a gourmet cook. I got my old singing coach back. When friends came to the house for a cocktail party, they said it was like night and day because I had changed so much. They saw me as a completely different person—more calm, confident, outgoing and energetic, and much more able to cope with everything. At times I wondered if I was getting too high, since this new personality, this new self, was foreign to me. In fact, it was the real me, which I had almost forgotten, because the depression had gone on for so many years. Although my friends thought that I had become transformed on Prozac, my husband—who had known me since I was in college—said that I had simply become the person I used to be."

For K.S., Prozac proved to be a miracle drug, but it has not enabled her to solve all her problems. Nonetheless, her spirits lifted dramatically. She is once again productive and creative, and her relationships with others have greatly improved. "My husband, strangely enough, does much more for me now than ever before," she noted. "Prozac has enabled me to shift away from depression, anxiety, and hopelessness and to move toward my previous more vivacious, energetic self. After ten years of depression, I'm delighted to be back."

In a sense, K.S. is an unusual case. Perhaps 90% of the patients who respond to Prozac will experience less dramatic results. They do not undergo anything even vaguely like a transformation. They simply come out of their depression. They get better.

Perhaps 10% of those who do respond to Prozac show an extraordinary reaction. Like K.S., these people are often misdiagnosed by physicians, therapists, and psychiatrists as suffering from anxiety neurosis, chronic depression, dysthymia or personality disorder. In fact, the patient has had a history of very mild to major manic depressive moodswings, ranging from those of the highly energetic, effective, slightly revved-up personalities to those with a family history of psychotic, hospitalized, suicidal, or manic depressive relatives. A physician who prescribes Prozac without recognizing the sometimes hidden elated or manic side of the patient's experience or heritage might expect only a gradual alleviation of symptoms—not a sudden, sometimes dangerous, transformation. With this information, the physician should be able to predict the usual antidepressant response as well as the spectacular and immediate change that can occur. Without taking a detailed family history, which in K.S.'s situation showed manic-depressive illness in the family and an energetic, driving personality in her own past, the physician is unprepared for the dramatic turn-around experienced by someone like her. These transformations are not mysterious. They are simply the reactions that I and other psychopharmacologists over the past thirty years have repeatedly seen in a small percentage of patients who have a personal or family history of moodswings ranging from depression to elation. These patients will respond rapidly and dramatically to any antidepressant drug and especially to Prozac and other similar drugs. (Some responders turn out to be manic depressives who also require lithium.)

This is why Prozac is such an exciting addition to psychopharmacology. In certain patients, many of whom have been unresponsive to previous antidepressant drugs, it dispels the bleak miasma of depression, revealing not a new, made-over version of the self but the original personality. In the case of K.S., a highly energetic personality emerged, one that had been hidden so long that both patient and friends had forgotten it existed.

If too high a dose of Prozac is given to a patient with a history similar to K.S.'s, the result may be more than a transformation; it may lead to manic psychosis. In these cases, a patient who was predisposed to experiencing strong highs and lows could have a reaction that physicians *might* call "Prozac toxic." This is not in fact toxicity but a full-blown manic state. To avoid this reaction, patients like K.S. must be given Prozac cautiously, in very low doses, and under the careful continuous monitoring of an expert psychiatrist or psychopharmacologist. Almost always, with severe manic-depressive patients, the addition of Lithium or one of its alternatives (Tegretol or Depakote) is necessary to avoid precipitating a full-blown manic state.

When patients like these are given Prozac in appropriate doses, they may appear to everyone to have undergone a spectacular metamorphosis. More often, it is simply the original personality, emerging at last out of the fog. The telltale signs and symptoms that act as predictors of this transformation can be found in the personal or family history. Most people don't experience this transformation. They just get well. With Prozac, they can look forward to a better, more fulfilling life—the life they were meant to lead.

What is Prozac?

Prozac is the first of a new class of antidepressant compounds called selective serotonin reuptake inhibitors, or SSRIs. Hailed as a miracle drug by millions of patients and numerous psychiatrists, trumpeted on the covers of magazines such as *Newsweek* ("a breakthrough drug for depression") and *New York* ("a new wonder drug"), and made notorious by the Church of Scientology's attacks, Prozac has become the best-selling antidepressant of all time. Its generic name is fluoxetine hydrochloride.

For what conditions is Prozac usually prescribed?

Prozac is usually prescribed for clinical or major depression, which along with its minor form, dysthymia, causes as many as 15 million Americans each year to feel sad, anxious, empty, and hopeless; to lose interest in life and enjoyment of its pleasures; to experience difficulty sleeping, eating, and concentrating in a normal way; to feel agitated or slowed down; and often to dwell on thoughts of death or suicide. Clinical trials of more than eleven thousand patients have clearly established Prozac as an effective medication for these mood disorders. In addition, the U.S. Food and Drug Administration has given Prozac its unanimous approval as a treatment for obsessive compulsive disorder.

Psychiatrists including myself have also used Prozac successfully in treating other varieties of depression, including atypical depression, the less severe long-lasting disorder known as minor depression or dysthymia, and, in combination with lithium, the down phase of manic depression.

An expanding array of other illnesses including bulimia, obesity, borderline personality, substance abuse, and other conditions appears to be responsive to Prozac based on a few scientific reports and many anecdotally reported individual cases. Although a limited number of positive reports of its usefulness in these conditions have been published, scientific studies have not yet been carried out in sufficient number, and the use of Prozac has not been FDA-approved for these conditions.

What about the claim that treatment of personality disorder with Prozac may cause complete transformations?

Claims like these lead inevitably to disappointment for most patients, although transformation does occur in a chosen few. Even on Prozac, shy depressives with personalities like that of the poet Emily Dickinson—unless they have a history of extreme highs and lows or family history of mood disorders—would not turn into extroverted rock and roll singers.

For most people, the changes created by Prozac are more subtle: the depression clears, the symptoms disappear, and positive life changes occur. A few of my patients who report feeling like themselves again say that they can't imagine living without Prozac. Indeed, it can offer a certain brightening, a new equanimity, or a boost in self-confidence. However, in patients who have major depression, this is a phenomenon that also occurs with most other antidepressant drugs.

Prozac is not a magic wand: seldom does it turn a wallflower into the belle of the ball. Nonetheless, like other psychiatrists, I have witnessed a few transformations and my interpretation of why they happen and how they can be predicted may surprise both patients and physicians.

What do people mean by personality transformation? And does Prozac transform personality?

Personality transformation as a result of taking Prozac is a concept articulated most strongly by the psychiatrist Peter D. Kramer, M.D., author of the best-selling book, *Listening to Prozac.* "Prozac seems to give confidence to the habitually timid, to make the sensitive brash, to lend the introvert the social skills of a salesman," he wrote. He pointed out that "Not all patients on Prozac respond this way. Some are unaffected by the medicine; some merely recover from depression, as they might on any antidepressant. But a few, a substantial minority, are transformed."

That concept swept the country. A number of psychiatrists reported individual cases of transformation, and magazines and newspapers further publicized it, referring to Prozac as a personality pill. Yet in my experience, transformation is extremely rare, something experienced not by a "substantial" minority but by a very small minority—at best no more than 10% of those patients who respond favorably to the drug.

Where the psychiatrists and I may differ is in the meaning of "transformation" and in the importance of a patient's genetic history.

There's no question that psychotropic drugs of all kinds, including anti-anxiety drugs, mood stabilizers, tranquilizers, and antidepressants, have the power to transform. When you change an individual's mood, lifting a person out of a depression (or calming down someone who is experiencing a manic high), that person's emotions, behavior, and even motor activity alter right along with the mood. A person who is less depressed becomes by definition livelier, more hopeful, and more energetic. It might sound like a transformation, but most patients don't experience it that way. "Prozac did not change my personality," one of my patients told me. "What Prozac has done for me is that it has lifted the black cloud of depression which so impaired my true personality and rendered me incapable of coping with my situation. My coping mechanism is now back intact along with my original personality—the one that can work efficiently and laugh as well as cry."

This is an important change, no question about it. But to label it a transformation is, in my view, to romanticize it and ignores the widely known genetic studies in this field. The reality is that all depressives, once they have returned to their normal state of mind, will say that they feel better about themselves and are more outgoing, efficient, and assertive. All antidepressant drugs can achieve those results. This is not news. Similarly, when depressed people with the propensity toward manic and hypomanic periods take antidepressant drugs, they tend to feel a greater sense of well-being than those without that propensity. And, because they are often dramatic, rejection-sensitive, histrionic personalities who magnify the elements of their lives, they make persuasive claims. They don't just feel better, they will tell you that with Prozac, they feel better than they've ever felt in their lives.

This is not news either, although the media has made it seem so. To thousands of experienced psychopharmacologists around the world, this has been articulated for at least thirty years in scientific journals and at conferences. As a group, these patients are hyperresponders who respond to all antidepressants and stimulants. And sooner or later, with every antidepressant that we've had, some of them slip into manic psychosis and end up in the hospital.

A few cases nonetheless appear to offer a stronger case for transformation, partially because these patients will waltz into the office on the very next visit and announce that they have been transformed. And indeed, the change is often dramatic. These patients are not merely lifted out of depression; they are elated. It is my contention that in the overwhelming number of cases, the reason for this so-called transformation is that these patients—often rapid responders—have always had a dual nature; they are sometimes depressed—sometimes for years on end—and they are sometimes, perhaps not as frequently, revved up. They are, in short, subtly bipolar. These are not full-blown manic-depressives; but they do have a family history of or a mild tendency toward the elevated moods of hyperthymia, hypomania, or cyclothymia. Prozac—or any other antidepressant, often enough—will nudge them into the manic zone—a place they have been before. Once there, they feel very, very good. And they will tell you so in vivid, dramatic language. But is this a transformation? If you think of the patient as a depressive, it may appear to be. If you think of the patient as a soft bipolar, it is not. It is indeed the predictable response that I and others who have studied the genetics of mood swings consistently see with our patients—a response that needs to be very carefully monitored.

How does Prozac compare with other drugs?

Despite its wonder drug label, Prozac is not the first successful antidepressant. Many psychiatrists, patients, and families have remarked upon Prozac's ability to enhance the patient's outlook, energy level, and mood, but the truth is that many other medications work just as well as Prozac in countering the effects of depression. For instance, in clinical scientific studies, Prozac and other antidepressants have a similar rate of success and a similar onset of action (one to two weeks for most people, although in many cases up to six weeks may need to pass before symptoms are relieved). Although carefully controlled studies of more than one or two years have not been completed, early reports suggest that Prozac, the other SSRIs, and Effexor are as effective in preventing depressive relapses in recurrent or unipolar depression as are the classic tricyclic antidepressants used over the last thirty years, such as amitriptyline (Elavil), imipramine (Tofranil), desipramine (Norpramine) and nortriptyline (Pamelor). It is also my impression that, when combined with lithium, Prozac appears to be effective in preventing relapses in patients with unipolar recurrent depression or bipolar manic depression.

The major difference between Prozac and other antidepressants is that Prozac is the first of a completely new category of antidepressant compounds, the SSRIs, all of which have minimal side effects. In addition, most patients receiving Prozac have to take only one capsule a day compared to previous antidepressants that require between three and six a day.

When and by whom was Prozac discovered?

Prozac was developed in 1972 by Bryan B. Molloy, David T. Wong, Ray W. Fuller, and other research scientists employed by Eli Lilly and Company. Clinical trials began in 1976. In December 1986, Prozac was marketed in Belgium, and one year later the U.S. Food and Drug Administration approved it for marketing in the United States. It caught on immediately. Between 1988 and 1989, the sales of Prozac almost tripled, going from $125 million to $350 million, and by 1990, it had become the most frequently prescribed antidepressant on the world market. The sale of Prozac, which by 1993 had reached $1 billion a year, has far exceeded the sale of all previously used antidepressant drugs on the American and world markets.

Who takes Prozac?

You'd be amazed. Since its introduction, over 11 million patients worldwide and 6 million in the United States have taken Prozac. These people cover the gamut from children to adolescents to the elderly, from lifelong depressives who, with the help of Prozac, are beginning for the first time to structure their lives in responsible ways, to many highly successful, productive people who have had from one to numerous bouts of depression in their lifetime. Name any randomly chosen group of successful people in society, business, politics, or the arts, and it is likely that 20% to 30% of them are either taking Prozac or have been given Prozac at some point over the last several years. Actors, politicians, housewives, businesspeople, and artists have flooded talk shows, newspapers, magazines, and books with stories of how Prozac has helped them. People of all classes, races, and religions have benefited from and talked about the miraculous effects of Prozac in reversing their despair, chronic lack of pleasure, poor functioning, and persistent low-level depression— and in raising them to a level of functioning so much better than their previous state that patients have sometimes used the term "new self."

In the past, lithium and other antidepressants have also unleashed a torrent of dramatic claims and testimony in books, articles, and talk shows. But, after media reports about the possibility of transforming the self and developing a new personality, Prozac has caused a deluge like no other. Prozac is so ubiquitous that, no matter where you live in the United States, you probably know someone who is taking it or has taken it.

Why do so many people take Prozac?

Prozac is a member of a new class of antidepressants with a different mechanism of action than previous antidepressant drugs. Although equal to past antidepressants in effectiveness, it is uniquely not lethal in overdose, nor is it toxic to the cardiovascular system compared to the older drugs. It is also easier to take, since its side effects are so much milder.

A lot of patients walk in *asking* for Prozac, whether they need it or not. Prozac has received more publicity than any other previously used psychiatric drug in America and abroad, and this unprecedented media attention has helped catapult Prozac to its current level of popularity. Seldom in the past did anyone I met at a dinner party question me about Tofranil or Nardil (although they did ask many times about lithium when its effectiveness as a treatment for manic depression first became known to the media). Now people ask about Prozac. Unlike other drugs, many of which are equally effective, Prozac has become a well-known, frequently requested remedy. Just as the most medically untutored know that a headache can be cured with aspirin, people who feel a little down today or want a personality "lift" are quick to discover that friends, family and the local GP have a single recommendation: Prozac. Sad to say, the media have oversold Prozac to the general public and to psychiatrists and other doctors. In my experience and in the experience of many of America's leading psychopharmacologists, the myth of Prozac's ability to cause a total personality metamorphosis has, more often than not, led to disappointment.

What percentage of patients who are taking Prozac are really helped by it?

Approximately 65% to 70% of depressed patients who take Prozac find that their symptoms are fully relieved within two to six weeks and that they are able to function normally once again. The other 30% to 35% of patients who don't respond or who can't tolerate the early side effects of nausea or insomnia that may occur for a couple of days in the beginning may respond instead to one of the older antidepressants; they may fall into the category of treatment-resistant (to all antidepressants); or they may respond to one of the new antidepressants such as Zoloft, Paxil, Effexor, Netazadone or an antidepressant still being tested in research clinical trials and not yet on the market.

The other well-tried older antidepressants have similar rates of success, but side effects are almost always present and bothersome.

How effective is Prozac in long-term prevention of depression and other diagnostic entities?

Although a sufficient number of carefully controlled long-term scientific studies of Prozac in recurrent depression have not been completed, early scientific reports, observations, and case histories from individual psychiatrists including myself have suggested that Prozac is as effective as earlier antidepressants in preventing the reappearance of depression, which usually returns in cycles. To keep this from happening, Prozac, like the other antidepressants, must be given on a long-term basis.

Can Prozac be used in children and adolescents?

Although scientific research in this area is scanty and incomplete, the evidence so far indicates that children and adolescents can safely be given Prozac, assuming that the dosage is small and is escalated slowly. Younger patients can be given small doses of liquid Prozac, while adolescents can probably take larger regular capsular doses approaching those of adults.

However, some evidence suggests that even in their late teens and early twenties, young people may do better with smaller doses. One limited study observed the reactions of fifteen depressed, treatment-resistant young people between 16 and 24 years old to being treated with Prozac for six or seven weeks. Although they were initially put on a standard dose of 20 mg of Prozac a day or even every other day, the dose was soon reduced to 5 or 10 mg a day. For a third of the patients, that small dose was enough to create a significant shift in the depression, which suggests that young people normally might be started on 5 or 10 mg a day.

Overall, seven of the eleven patients who completed this study showed a positive change according to one standard depression rating scale, and eight showed significant improvement according to another scale. Considering that these young people had been unsuccessfully treated with other antidepressants, this admittedly small study offers real hope.

However, it is absolutely essential that the prescribing physician take a detailed family history, which can reveal a genetic predisposition toward manic depression. In some cases, children taking Prozac have become agitated, and one published study described five adolescent girls, all with family histories riddled with major depression and suicide, who developed mania while taking Prozac. This is not at all surprising to me, since the family histories also revealed evidence of manic depression or one of its genetically linked illnesses such as alcohol and drug abuse, suicide, gambling, depression, or sociopathy.

The need still exists for carefully controlled clinical studies comparing the responses of children and adolescents to Prozac and other standard drugs. In the meantime, youngsters taking Prozac should be observed closely and frequently, and side effects should be reported. If the psychiatrist or the family is in doubt about the child's response or any emerging side effects, the drug should be discontinued. A child psychopharmacologist who specializes in treating childhood depression with drugs is the most appropriate person to consult.

Can Prozac be safely used in the elderly who are depressed?

This is an important question, because depression hits the elderly hard. Depression is four times more common among the elderly than in the general population, and the suicide rate for people over 65 is fifteen times greater than that of the overall population.

The early studies of Prozac in the elderly go back to 1985. Open studies and double blind studies indicate that Prozac relieves the symptoms of depression just as well as other antidepressants in geriatric patients. Certainly, mild doses of nortriptyline (Aventyl or Pamelor) have been successful in elderly depressed patients in the opinion of many psychiatrists, and other psychiatrists may swear by any number of the older drugs as highly effective. However, patients taking Prozac complained less frequently of dry mouth and constipation, which are typically reported with other antidepressant drugs, and they were much less likely to drop out of the study due to adverse effects. Prozac also lacks adverse cardiovascular effects, compared to the tricyclic antidepressants, and is much less dangerous when taken in overdose. In the opinion of most psychopharmacologic experts, Prozac or one of the other SSRIs is the preferred antidepressant in the elderly.

Does Prozac cure depression or any other illnesses for which it is given?

The concept of "cure," so basic for physicians with other specialties, is an elusive one for psychiatrists. Prozac does not cure depression or any other chronic or recurrent illness for which it is prescribed; thus, it is similar to all other psychotropic drugs that alleviate illness but do not cure it. From 75% to 80% of depressed patients have depression that tends to recur.

On the other hand, Prozac and other antidepressants sometimes appear to cure. Perhaps 20% to 25% of the patients whose depression is relieved by Prozac or other medications are never destined to have a recurrence. This does not mean that the illness has been cured by the antidepressant drug, although it certainly looks that way. Rather, the patient was destined through genetics and environment to have only one depressive episode in his or her lifetime.

Why has Prozac been featured on the covers of *Newsweek* **and** *New York Magazine,* **discussed on major television and radio stations, and written about in most of the daily newspapers in this country?**

The sensational press coverage that Prozac has received is due partly to the growing public awareness of depression over the past two decades. Educational programs sponsored by groups such as the American Psychiatric Association, the National Depressive and Manic-Depression Association, and my own Foundation for Depression and Manic Depression in New York City, have helped broadcast the message locally and nationally that depression is a physical illness that can be treated quickly and effectively with antidepressants. Powerful memoirs such as the actress Patty Duke's *A Brilliant Madness: Living with Manic-Depressive Illness* and the author William Styron's *Darkness Visible* have shed light on an emotion that Winston Churchill described as a "black cloud" and that one of my own patients called a "black hole." And a flurry of interest in depression always rises up in the wake of events such as the 1993 suicide of President Bill Clinton's boyhood friend and White House legal adviser Vincent Foster.

This increased public awareness has improved the climate for talking about and dealing with major depression. A patient of mine for twenty years, now in her seventies, who has been coping with recurrent bouts of depression for half a century, told me, "When you break a leg, you talk about it. When it's your nerves, you don't." This is changing. When imipramine, the first antidepressant, was discovered in 1958, no one talked about depression. By the time Prozac was introduced in 1987, that taboo had largely evaporated.

In addition to its promised ability to alleviate depression, Prozac's "mood enhancing" or "mood brightening" properties caught the attention of the public and the media. Its effects were presented as dramatic and miraculous—and, let's face it, a lot of people in our culture continue to look for a quick fix. Unfortunately, the newspaper and magazine articles and talk shows failed to delineate the myth from the reality and did not make the point that major transformations, when they did occur, took place in perhaps 10% of Prozac responders. The media instead implied that most everyone, depressed or not, who even has a few personality quirks might take Prozac and have complete relief of all unpleasant symptoms as well as a personality change. It was heralded that slower going, somewhat introspective, chronically unhappy people, upon taking Prozac, could become upbeat, highly confident, energetic, extroverted people. They would essentially be able to change their personalities to what the American culture considers most desirable—the highly energized and charismatic personality with the competitive edge. Then, in the middle of all this media attention, came an all-out attack orchestrated by the Church of Scientology. It focused on a very small group of people, among the millions who have taken Prozac, who had suicidal or violent thoughts or in a few instances actually committed suicide or homicide. These rare cases led the press and the media to produce more coverage on the possibly negative effects of the drug, charges of which Prozac was later exonerated. All in all, Prozac has received more than its share of publicity, both good and bad.

• 2 •

Depression, the Manic-Depressive Spectrum, and Unrecognized Mood Disorders

The concept of depression has entered the public's consciousness so fully that many people today use the word "depressed" in the same way that they might once have described themselves as dejected, discouraged, or simply glum. At the same time, many people who believe they are in a *temporary* down or think they are reacting in a normal, healthy way to difficult circumstances are in fact clinically depressed and should seek both diagnosis and treatment.

Clinical depression does not simply go away. Depression is worse than unhappiness, more than malaise, and not in the least like a stubborn refusal to "buck up." In the psychiatrist's lexicon, "depression" is a term that can be applied to a collection of disorders, each of which is characterized by a constellation of specific and debilitating symptoms. It is not a monolithic disorder. Just as major (or clinical) depression is not the same as simply feeling down, major depression is also not the same as minor depression (now categorized by psychiatrists as dysthymia). Likewise, feeling manic is not the same as feeling happy.

The questions in this chapter concern two main topics: the many varieties of depression and its "nonidentical twin sister" elation; and the impact of Prozac and other drugs in its class upon these many mood disorders characterized mainly by depression—but also by subtle to shockingly obvious states of manic elation.

What is major depression?

According to the fourth edition of the American Psychiatric Association's *Diagnostic and Statistical Manual of Mental Disorders (DSM-IV)*, a typical episode of major depressive disorder lasts at least two weeks and includes most (but not necessarily all) of the following symptoms:

- a low mood: feeling sad, empty, despondent
- loss of interest in life
- the inability to find pleasure in activities that used to be enjoyable, including sex
- weight loss or weight gain
- trouble sleeping or excess sleeping
- feelings of hopelessness, helplessness, guilt, and worthlessness
- trouble concentrating and making decisions
- lack of energy
- anxiety
- feelings of agitation or of having slowed down
- frequent thoughts about death, self-destructive ideas, or the feeling of not wanting to live.

Some people experience these symptoms once in their lives, while others suffer from repeated bouts of major depression. This much is certain: depression is widespread. According to one estimate, at any given moment, about one person in twenty is grappling with depression, and over the course of a lifetime, one person in ten will have at least one episode of major depression.

Is there more than one kind of depression?

Yes. Here are some of the types that fall under the category of primary depression:

- Major depression, also known as unipolar or clinical depression, is a disorder that is usually recurrent, with repeated depressive episodes alternating with normal periods.

- Dysthymia is a type of depression in which symptoms are relatively mild but present most of the time and persistent for at least two years.

- Manic-depressive (bipolar I) disorder is characterized by dark periods of moderate to severe depression alternating with manic highs, which are often severe enough to require hospitalization.

- Manic-depressive (bipolar II) disorder involves periods of major depression interspersed with mildly manic—or hypomanic—episodes, which are usually pleasurable or irritable in nature.

Cyclothymia is the mildest form of manic depression, alternating periods of hypomania and dysthymia. In the depressed phases of these categories, one may see either agitation, in which the depression is accompanied by a collection of frantic symptoms such as difficulty sitting still, insomnia, and loss of appetite, or retardation, in which movements, speech, and other responses are slowed down and the patient tends to sleep and eat too much.

Psychiatrists use the term "secondary depression" when depression is secondary to a medical or other primary psychiatric disorder, such as general anxiety disorder, panic disorder, substance abuse, sleep disorder, or schizophrenia. It is occasionally linked with a few medically prescribed drugs, some of which are associated with the onset of depression (particularly antihypertensives). Steroids, amphetamines, and Ritalin may be associated with the onset of secondary mania and hypomania.

The term "normal reactive depression" describes the grief experienced by people who are mourning a loss.

Finally, a few disorders slip between the cracks and are consequently classified in the *DSM-IV* under the official phrase "Not Otherwise Specified." (*See Glossary*). Examples include recurrent brief depressive disorder and premenstrual dysphoric disorder.

For what kinds of depression is Prozac most commonly given?

Prozac is only approved in the United States for major depressive disorder and obsessive-compulsive disorder. Nevertheless, psychiatrists have also commonly used it for a wide range of other diagnoses, including dysthymia, atypical bipolar depression, the depressive phase of bipolar manic depression, borderline personality disorder, substance abuse, several other personality disorders and subclinical forms of depression. (See below for further discussion of each of these diagnoses.) In addition, Prozac appears to be effective for bulimia.

It is also used with some reported efficacy in instances where the depression is secondary to a primary medical or psychiatric illness such as panic disorder, phobic disorder, or even obesity.

What is the difference between feeling blue and being depressed?

Almost everyone at one point or another experiences *normal* depression, a brief period of joyless, dejected, sad feelings that can accompany the usual day-to-day vicissitudes of life. In that sense, feeling blue or down in the dumps can be a normal reaction to disappointing life events if it is short-lived and transitory, lasting perhaps as little as an hour or, at most, a day or two. Once the adverse events are resolved or the person has had the chance to adapt to changed circumstances, the feeling of being down or blue usually evaporates on its own. And in the meantime, the person continues to function.

Major depression is something else. It does not just blow away in the course of a week or ten days. It persists for at least two weeks, according to the *DSM-IV* criteria, and sometimes for years. On the average, a major depression lasts three to eight months. Because it lasts longer and is more serious than temporary feelings of lethargy, gloominess, or sadness, it impairs functioning in a real way.

Since the word "depression" is sometimes used to mean anything from a passing mood to a clinical illness, the first thing any doctor must do when a patient comes into the office and complains of feeling blue or depressed is to conduct a detailed psychiatric diagnostic evaluation, obtain a recent physical exam, and get a personal and family history. A patient who lacks sufficient symptoms to make a *DSM-IV* diagnosis of one of the depressive disorders may simply be experiencing a temporary down—a normal depression. Or the patient may be experiencing a subclinical depression with only one to two depressive symptoms. In the latter case, many psychiatrists, and particularly psychotherapists, term the subclinical depression a personality disorder since it does not meet the full *DSM-IV* criteria for any of the main categories of depression.

Prozac should not be used for the transitory down or unhappy feelings that everyone at times experiences. These are part of our normal range of emotions.

On the other hand, if the depression lasts for more than a few weeks, and is accompanied by a sufficient number of *DSM-IV* symptoms, a diagnosis of major depression, dysthymia, or bipolar depression is made and action in the form of medication needs to be taken by a trained expert. This is usually a psychiatrist specifically trained in giving medications (psychopharmacologist).

What's the difference between anxiety and depression?

Anxiety is an uneasy feeling of worry, apprehension, and distress, often about the future. Psychiatrists sometimes distinguish between anxiety, which can be thought of as a reaction to an ambiguous or imagined danger, and fear, which is a response to a real threat.

Depression, especially as laypersons use the term, is a bleak mood typically characterized by discouragement, sadness, or despair. In a sense, anxiety, with its finger-drumming restlessness, and depression, with its hopeless inertia, are quite different, which is why psychiatrists classify anxiety disorders separately from depressive disorders. Yet the two feeling states so frequently overlap and co-exist that the difference between anxiety and depressive disorders is confusing. The primary diagnosis is based on the answer to a simple question: in the life history of the patient, which state did the patient experience first?

Thus, in anxiety disorders, anxiety is the primary symptom and often the first symptom, even though frequently secondary depression is present. Anxiety disorders include:

- general anxiety disorder
- phobic disorder
- panic disorder
- obsessive-compulsive disorder
- post-traumatic stress disorder (PTSD).

In depressive disorders, the depressed mood usually appears first as the primary symptom and is normally the most important part of the illness. However, although anxiety is not always present in depressive disorders, most of the time it lurks beneath the surface in varying degrees and may be present as one of a number of symptoms within the depressive syndrome.

Does Prozac treat both anxiety and depression? One of them better than the other?

Most of the scientific investigations of Prozac have focused on depression, with the result that Prozac has received FDA approval for use in major depression. It has not been approved for anxiety disorders because enough data haven't been accumulated from scientifically conducted trials. Furthermore, from the data so far, the trend may not support using Prozac for primary anxiety disorders.

Nevertheless, when patients suffering from major depression and the milder form dysthymia are treated with Prozac, symptoms of anxiety typically lift along with the other symptoms of depression. To date, a limited number of studies indicate that

Prozac does not seem to be useful for General Anxiety Disorder (GAD) but it is therapeutic for panic attacks and the secondary anxiety seen in major depressive disorders and dysthymia. Once the depression is relieved, the secondary disorder tends to disappear as well.

What is dysthymia?

Dysthymia, a term coined in the 1980s for minor depression, was previously known in the 1950s as depressive neurosis and in the 1970s as depressive personality. It is a mild but persistent form of depression that afflicts at least 2 to 3 million people. According to the *DSM-IV* criteria, a diagnosis of dysthymia requires a patient to have been depressed most of the time for at least two years (one year for children and adolescents). In addition, at least three of the following symptoms must be present:

- low self-esteem or lack of confidence
- pessimism, hopelessness, or despair
- lack of interest in ordinary pleasures and activities
- withdrawal from social activities
- fatigue or lethargy
- guilt or ruminating about the past
- irritability or excessive anger
- lessened productivity
- difficulty concentrating or making decisions.

Because the symptoms of dysthymia are less severe than those of major depression, dysthymia is not always recognized and is sometimes misdiagnosed as a personality disorder. The importance of the diagnosis cannot be underestimated because diagnosis determines treatment. Yet in psychiatry, diagnosis can be imprecise. Psychotic hallucinations, for instance, can be a symptom of schizophrenia, which is notoriously difficult to treat, or of severe manic depression, which can be controlled with lithium. Unhappiness and feelings of emptiness can be characteristic of borderline personality disorder or of dysthymia. The difference is major. If the diagnosis is dysthymia, medications such as Prozac may help. We have treatments. If the diagnosis is a personality disorder, the treatment involves many years of therapy, and the prognosis is guarded. Thus, if a patient is diagnosed as having a disease which he or she does not have, or for which there is no cure, then nothing will be done to help the patient. In this sense, whether you get well or not is determined by the diagnosis. The importance of finding an experienced doctor is critical because the diagnosis—along with the doctor's knowledge of which drug to choose and in what dosage—can determine the person's fate.

A patient of mine, E.R., was referred to me by a psychologist who had treated him in psychotherapy for over two years for a "personality disorder." During this time, there was little or no response to treatment. After reading numerous articles in newspapers and magazines that described remarkable improvements in patients that sounded exactly like this one, the psychologist finally decided to send him to me for a psychopharmacology consultation. E.R. reported in the initial interview that for four or five years, even though he functioned as an engineer and was successfully married with children, he had not felt like his normal self and was only going through the motions of life with very little pleasure, often in a slight daze and in slow motion. After a physical exam and a careful psychiatric evaluation along with a family history, I diagnosed him as suffering from chronic dysthymia and began treating him with Prozac. Within three weeks, he reported to me that Prozac had made a dramatic difference and had changed his mood "from chronic pessimism to optimism. It has been a miracle drug for me," he states. "I am a different person—and everyone around me agrees, especially my wife and family." Although his long-term mild dysthymia by definition had never been severe, the persistence of this low-grade depressive mood disorder had affected all aspects of his living. Although he was "getting along OK professionally" and had managed to establish a family, he had simply never had the normal energy and zest for life that he now seems to feel with Prozac.

What is bipolar manic depression? Hypomania?

Bipolar manic depression is a disorder characterized by periods of major depression alternating with periods of elevated mood. When those periods of elation are severe, they are known as mania and the diagnosis is bipolar I. When the periods of elation are relatively mild, or hypomanic, the diagnosis is bipolar II. About 25% of the people who experience major depression also experience these periods of high, and the contrast between the two poles (hence the term "bipolar") is dramatic. Hypomanic patients become overactive socially, physically, and sexually. Characteristically tireless in energy, they may be garrulous and expansive, charming, and irritable or angry, and they are often seductive at the office, cracking risqué jokes. During a full manic episode, into which the hypomanic state sometimes grows, the increased energy is extreme. People experiencing this manic state may literally go for two or three days without sleep at all. Hypomanic people, who usually require only four or five hours of sleep, are constantly busy, talking, telephoning, faxing, planning, and implementing numerous schemes. Hypomanic women in the home are often described as "super moms." Everyone tends to admire hypomaniacs except when they seem to lose judgment or snap back angrily when their opinion is challenged or when they are crossed. Their minds often race, and they periodically overestimate their own abilities. Their judgment in politics, business, and the arts may be extremely sharp. Yet at other times their judgment is poor. As the hypomanic mood develops, at times coming dangerously close to a full mania, they may take irresponsible risks, drive recklessly, go on spending sprees, or participate in a multitude of sexual liaisons.

In the most severe form of the illness, manic-depressive patients become psychotic. Those who experience four or more mood swings a year are referred to as rapid cycling manic depressives.

Even though patients often use the word "high" to describe these hypomanic or manic episodes, the mood in many cases is not euphoric but irritable, paranoid, and angry, leading to confrontations and rage attacks. In its most severe form, known as psychotic mania, the manic-depressive patient may hallucinate or have grandiose religious or paranoid delusions. Because manic patients seldom perceive that they are ill, they often refuse to see psychiatrists or take any medication. However, if severe mania is left untreated, there is a risk of full psychosis and collapse brought on by physical and mental exhaustion. Hospitalization is usually required to prevent harm to themselves or others. Often, this hospitalization must be made at the request of the family, and, unfortunately, it must occasionally be legally forced when two psychiatrists deem that the patient presents a threat to him or herself or to others in the community.

How is manic depression treated?

Many manic depressives are treated with lithium alone, which helps smooth out the rough hills and valleys of the emotional landscape. (In some cases, if lithium cannot be tolerated or is simply ineffective, antiepileptic medications Tegretol or Depakote have been used to stabilize mood and behavior.) Often, however, lithium isn't enough. The mania may be controlled, but the periods of depression are still too numerous and too deep. In about 30% of the cases, when the lows are not fully controlled even with lithium, the intermittent or permanent addition of an antidepressant may be called for. Before Prozac and other SSRIs became available, psychiatrists used almost every antidepressant drug on the market in combination with lithium. Now increasing successes have been reported with the combination of lithium and Prozac. Many manic depressives use both drugs simultaneously for an indefinite period of time. Others may need both drugs to get over a single depressive episode, but if the attacks recur while the patient's on lithium alone, Prozac and lithium in combination can be used successfully on a long-term maintenance basis. Prozac should not be given to severe bipolar I manic depressives without lithium and/or other mood stabilizers, since it may make the manic high dangerously higher, requiring hospitalization for manic psychosis. Even with antimanic medications, manic breakthroughs and toxic drug reactions have occasionally been reported with Prozac and other SSRIs.

What is the difference between mania and hypomania?

The difference is basically one of degree. The *DSM-IV* defines hypomania as "a distinct period of sustained elevated, expansive, or irritable mood, lasting throughout four days." Mania is a longer, more intense version of the same thing. The manic mood is not just elevated but "abnormally and persistently elevated," and it lasts at least one week—twice as long as a hypomanic episode.

In addition, a person in a manic or hypomanic state would be expected to have at least three of the following symptoms:

- excessive self-esteem or grandiosity
- reduced need for sleep
- extreme talkativeness, excessive telephoning
- extremely rapid flight of thoughts along with the feeling that the mind is racing
- inability to concentrate, easily distracted
- increase in social or work-oriented activities, often with a sixty- to eighty-hour work week
- poor judgment, as indicated by misguided business decisions, sprees of uncontrolled spending, or an increase in sexual indiscretions.

Again, the difference between mania and hypomania is one of degree. While both states might be described using terms such as those listed, hypomania can simply seem like a more productive, active period, whereas a full-blown manic attack seriously impairs functioning and often requires hospitalization. Manic people are out of control: they can hurt themselves and others. But those who are hypomanic can also exercise poor judgment. Some patients make excursions from a pleasurable (or sometimes irritable) hypomania to a shockingly destructive mania, affecting everyone and everything around them.

Can Prozac induce a manic high?

In patients inclined to be bipolar or manic-depressive, Prozac has been frequently reported to induce a manic or hypomanic state, which is why this drug must be prescribed and monitored with great care in such patients. This is a serious problem—and it is certainly something to watch carefully—but keep in mind that all antidepressants present the same danger. Since imipramine, the first antidepressant, was introduced in 1958, hypomanic highs have been induced by *every* antidepressant on the market, including the tricyclics, MAOIs (Monoamine Oxidase Inhibitors), the second generation antidepressants, the SSRIs, Wellbutrin and Effexor.

What is recurrent unipolar depression?

Unipolar depression is the same as major depression, which is the same as clinical depression. It is considered unipolar because, whereas manic depressives experience both terrible lows and manic highs (the twin poles of their disorder), people afflicted with unipolar depression only experience the down phase. When episodes happen repeatedly over the course of months or years, the illness is considered recurrent.

How common are the various types of depression?

About 3% to 4% of the population experiences major depression. Manic depression occurs in another 1% or 2%, and another 5% of the population suffers from one of the other forms of depression, including dysthymia, chronic treatment-resistant depression, and depression secondary to medical or other psychiatric disorders. All told, about 10% of the population is afflicted by depression in one form or another, with women about two to five times more likely than men to be affected. Manic depression, however, afflicts men and women equally.

What is cyclothymic disorder, and is Prozac good for it?

Cyclothymic disorder is a mild form of manic depression that for the most part goes untreated. Indeed, many depression experts consider both hypomanic and cyclothymic patients as highly useful and productive in the society. During the mild highs, these people feel extremely well and are often very productive, while the symptoms of depression in the cyclothymic patient seem to be simply periods of letdown, discouragement, and loss of productivity.

Cyclothymic disorder can be diagnosed after two years (one for children and adolescents) in which a patient who usually continues to function quite reasonably has had several hypomanic episodes along with numerous periods of depression. These ups and downs do not meet the full criteria for major depression. Between the mood swings the symptoms never disappear for longer than two months at a time. Yet there is no clear evidence of a major depressive or manic disorder. The ups are energetic and productive, while the downs are simply tolerable, with the person becoming more pessimistic and withdrawn. Cyclothymics usually remain cyclothymics, and they appear to be afflicted by mild versions of manic-depressive disorder. In some instances, however, the episode may change into full-blown manic depression. Manic depression requires treatment with lithium, and, in some instances, cyclothymia requires lithium treatment as well.

The use of Prozac in cyclothymia has not been adequately studied, but the very nature of the illness makes this an area for caution. Presumably, from all we know about Prozac, it would alleviate the depression. The problem is that it could also accentuate the periods of hypomania. Thus, it could conceivably turn a cyclothymic disorder into full-blown manic depression. For this reason, Prozac should not be used on a long-term basis in cyclothymic patients, and if used in the depressive phase, it should be used very cautiously, and in smaller doses than usual. However, if Prozac is given in conjunction with lithium or one of its alternatives, it could theoretically provide safe, long-term protection against the ups and downs of cyclothymia.

What is hyperthymia?

The term "hyperthymia" implies an energetic, confident, active, sometimes irritable but essentially normal personality type who is successfully balancing a multitude of projects and relationships. All of these personality traits (except the irritability) are considered highly desirable in Western culture.

A number of genetic studies including those undertaken by my own group indicate that people who are hyperthymic may come from a family in which manic-depressive relatives have struggled with depression, suicide, gambling, sociopathy, or alcohol or drug abuse. The family tree often has family members with hyperthymic or dysthymic personalities. Usually the manic-depressive pedigree includes one or more relatives who have been highly energetic, creative, and accomplished. If no major mood swings occur in this latter group of people, they are referred to simply as hyperthymic personalities. These individuals do not seek treatment since things are going well. For the most part, these are people who get things done in all walks of life. They either charm you or irritate you, but they usually produce.

What is subclinical depression?

Subclinical depression is depression that is not extensive enough in symptoms to merit a diagnosis of major depression or dysthymia according to *DSM-IV,* which categorizes various mental and emotional diseases and lists required symptoms for each major diagnostic category.

However, a patient diagnosed with a given disorder doesn't necessarily display every one of those listed characteristic symptoms. Of the nine symptoms listed for major depression, any five permit the diagnosis. Dysthymia also has a list of nine symptoms; only three are required for the diagnosis. A diagnosis of mania or hypomania also requires a specific number of symptoms, but mild hypomania, unlike mania, may cause little or no impairment of functioning and may be, in fact, desirable.

But what about patients who have only two of the traits needed for diagnosis of major depression? Or only one? Feelings of despair, hopelessness, and pessimism alone aren't enough to diagnose major depression or dysthymia. Merely feeling depressed, sad, empty, timid, or withdrawn most of the time does not qualify as major depression or dysthymia, although these are certainly a few of the symptoms included in these syndromes. Some patients, normal in all other respects, may only exhibit sleep disruption or a severe drop in self-esteem or a fear of new social situations. Other patients may come in with a myriad of physical complaints, none of which can be explained by physical causes, and alone these complaints do not allow the physician to diagnose depression.

Because these patients fall short of the totality of the required *DSM-IV* symptoms for diagnosing major depression or dysthymia, manifesting only a single, or a few isolated symptoms of the illness (depression) they, therefore, do not qualify for one of the *DSM-IV* diagnoses. Instead, they are counted among the *subclinically* depressed and are often exclusively treated in psychotherapy, either sitting or lying on the couch, by the psychoanalyst, psychologist, psychiatrist, or social work-therapist.

People who fall into this category often remain incompletely diagnosed and untreated because they may continue to function fairly well and don't feel enough pain to go to a psychiatrist. They may instead go to their internist or psychologist and be diagnosed with "irritable bowel syndrome" or "personality disorder." They're just miserable most of the time, and misery is not a formal psychiatric diagnosis.

Often considered ideal candidates for psychoanalysis, these patients have been called the "worried well." They tend to seek psychotherapy, feeling that their timidity, lack of interest, difficulty competing with their peers, and low self-confidence are psychological problems, which will be "cured" on the couch. When the subclinical depressive symptoms have been chronic, therapy alone usually fails. But I have seen many patients with subclinical depressions who have responded very well to Prozac, in combination with personal short-term psychotherapy.

What is meant by atypical depression?

In a usual depression, most people tend to lose weight and have difficulty sleeping, whereas the distinctive feature of atypical depression is that patients tend to gain weight and to sleep more than is normal. They also tend to be extremely anxious, histrionic, sensitive to rejection, and strongly reactive to environmental factors. Major depression typically does not have these latter symptoms.

The symptoms of atypical depression have traditionally responded best to Monoamine Oxidase Inhibitors, but studies now suggest that Prozac and probably other SSRIs may also be effective in treating this disorder.

What is double depression, and can Prozac be used to treat this condition?

Double depression is a diagnosis made when a patient who has been suffering from chronic, long-term mild depression (dysthymia) plummets into an episode of major depression. Many psychiatrists have found that maintaining a patient on Prozac seems both to treat the dysthymia and to prevent the superimposed major depression from recurring. Although no clear-cut studies have proven Prozac to be effective in double depression, psychiatrists have reported numerous case histories in which both forms of depression seem to be alleviated and even prevented by Prozac. Often the dosage must be increased when the major depression occurs on top of dysthymia.

What is chronic treatment-resistant depression?

When a depression is so persistent that it lasts over a year and so tenacious that it is unaffected by all major classes of antidepressants and therapies, it is classified as chronic and treatment-resistant. This is an area where Prozac, Zoloft, Paxil, and Effexor have provided some patients with a significant breakthrough. A number of chronically depressed individuals previously nonresponsive to antidepressant medications have been helped by Prozac and these newer drugs.

A 58-year-old married businessman, C.L., told me that he had been mildly depressed most of his life, a condition I diagnosed as chronic dysthymia. He also had had two severe depressions occurring at ages 28 and 31 so that at these times he really was suffering from double depression. C.L. had tried various kinds of talking and antidepressant drug therapies and had spent thousands of dollars, with little or no success. Finally, his wife persuaded him to give Prozac a try. After I reviewed his initial physical exam and electrocardiogram (EKG), which were normal, C.L. and I spent an hour discussing his past, present, and family psychiatric history. His family history revealed an uncle with major depression, a 20-year-old daughter who was having "personality problems" including mild depressive mood swings, and a brother who had committed suicide.

Putting all of this together, my diagnosis of C.L. was that he was suffering from chronic treatment-resistant depression, which on two occasions had developed into double depression. Neither the dysthymia nor the major depressions had ever had any sustained response to either psychotherapy or medications. After I explained the pros and cons of the newest antidepressant medications, he agreed to take Prozac, to be monitored by me and my staff weekly for the first month and, if substantial improvement occurred, to see me monthly thereafter.

After four weeks of Prozac, during which time the daily dosage was escalated from 10 to 40 mg, C.L. announced that his depression had been "pretty much eliminated." He had complained the first week of slight nausea and trouble getting to sleep, but he had stuck with it, and these side effects disappeared by the end of week two.

At week four, C.L. reported, "After all these years of getting nowhere with drugs and therapy, I am really grateful that I have found something that finally works." However, in his opinion he was not *transformed;* he still had complaints about his marriage and wanted to talk about them in psychotherapy.

Nonetheless, C.L. grudgingly rated his own mood as fairly normal for the first time in years.

It struck me that, after years of chronic irritability and mild depression most of the time, Prozac was essentially acting as a miracle drug for this patient. C.L. didn't admit to being transformed, but as his psychiatrist, I was amazed at his fabulous response. Over the years, I have treated other chronic treatment-resistant patients with other drugs, but I have seldom seen such a remarkable improvement.

What is secondary depression?

Secondary depression can develop in the presence of a previously existing condition, whether it is medical, such as a hypothyroidism, stroke, Parkinson's disease, or AIDS, or psychiatric, such as schizophrenia, panic disorder, or bulimia, among others. The key is which came first. When the depression clearly develops chronologically *after* the other primary medical or psychiatric condition, it is considered secondary.

Is Prozac an effective treatment for secondary depression?

It can be. But the first step should always be to focus on bringing the primary disorder under control. If the depression persists even after the primary illness has been treated, Prozac can be added and is often effective, as are other antidepressants.

Antidepressants can also be effective in the presence of other psychiatric disorders and can be combined with other medications, so long as the primary treatment is *not* an MAOI antidepressant. In the case of schizophrenia, Prozac can be safely combined with major tranquilizers. When anxiety disorders are primary, Prozac can be given with minor tranquilizers, and when the diagnosis is bipolar manic depres-

sion, it can be taken along with lithium, Tegretol, or
Depakote.

With obsessive-compulsive disorder, bulimia, and
panic disorder, evidence is emerging that Prozac
may alleviate the symptoms of both the primary
illness and the secondary depression so often experienced in these disorders.

What is a dysphoric mood?

A dysphoric mood is an unpleasant emotional
state with feelings of sadness, anxiety, and/or irritability. If short in duration, it is usually not severe
enough to lead to a major impairment of functioning.
Psychiatrists use the term to describe patients who
complain of a shifting set of symptoms. These mood
changes, if transitory, are often normal responses to
ordinary (but momentous) events of life such as
leaving home for the first time, falling in love, or
losing a loved one. Dysphoric moods can also accompany medical disorders such as stroke or Alzheimer's disease.

However, if the dysphoric mood swings become
prolonged for weeks or longer, the patient should be
evaluated. The dysphoria may evolve into a bona
fide depression, which needs to be treated.

What are the symptoms of grief or bereavement, and does Prozac help in its treatment?

We usually think of grief only in terms of the
death of a loved one, but bereavement reactions also
occur in response to the loss of a job, a large quan-
tity of money, an important object such as a home,
or even an idealistic concept that one has long pur-
sued. Weeping, anxiety, sadness, anger, irritability,
guilt, insomnia, and obsessive thinking about the
loss are all common reactions, but if these symptoms
do not begin to level off after three to four months,

psychiatrists usually diagnose major depressive disorder. In such cases, Prozac or another antidepressant, along with therapy, is indicated. Indeed, it may help earlier.

What does the term "masked depression" refer to, and can it be treated with Prozac?

Masked depression refers to depression that is hidden behind physical complaints for which no organic cause can be found. The physician's tendency is usually to dismiss these patients as hypochondriacs or to label them as anxious and prescribe minor tranquilizers to calm them down or stimulants to pep them up and get them out of the office as quickly as possible.

Masked depression (also known as depressive equivalent, latent depression, hidden depression, overlooked depression, or disguised depression) is potentially one of the most frustrating and therefore serious of mental disorders for the patient, since if not diagnosed correctly and treated properly, the patient is likely to "doctor hop" for years, trying the patience of one physician after another. As Freud himself noted, physical complaints can dominate the clinical picture and lead one to believe that the disorder is strictly physical rather than emotional. In these instances, a succession of M.D.s may never address the patient's despair. In the worst case, the patient will give up and commit suicide.

Since the underlying illness is depression, Prozac, like other antidepressants, can often be used effectively, although little research has been done on Prozac's effect on masked depression per se. Because the new antidepressants (of which Prozac, Zoloft, Paxil, and Effexor are examples) have fewer side effects, it is most likely that patients with masked depression will be responsive to these drugs as they have been to the older antidepressants. The critical issue is to make the correct diagnosis of depression, since it is hidden to the patient and often the doctor fails to detect it as well and attempts to treat it as a medical condition.

How common is suicide among the different subtypes of depression?

Even as underreported as it probably is, suicide is the eighth leading cause of death in the United States. Every year, roughly thirty thousand people kill themselves, and about eight to ten times that number make unsuccessful attempts. Suicide is more common among men (although women make four times as many attempts), those over 45, those who have never married or are divorced or widowed, those with chronic medical conditions, and, most significantly, those who have mood disorders. Most patients with major depression have suicidal thoughts at some time in their lives, and many of these patients carry out suicide attempts. A full 15% of those who suffer from repeated bouts of major depression ultimately kill themselves. Manic depressives are also prone to suicide, especially in the depressed phase of manic depression (16%). Some 10% of schizophrenics kill themselves, as do 5% of those with antisocial personality disorder. Drug addicts, prisoners, patients in mental hospitals, and people diagnosed with physical illnesses all have higher than normal suicide rates. Finally, alcoholics have a high rate of suicide, with as many as 15% ultimately killing themselves—and that's not counting the long, slow suicide that masks as cirrhosis, the seventh leading cause of death in the United States.

Is it justified to give Prozac to patients who are not suffering from an identifiable psychiatric illness but who have one or two symptoms?

Symptoms such as low self-esteem, sadness, sluggishness, or chronic discouragement may not add up to full-blown depression or dysthymia but can be considered symptoms of subclinical or subsyndromal depression, which is about to become a new diagnostic entity. In previous years, subclinical depression hadn't been identified as a formal *DSM* disorder. Instead, psychiatrists and analysts diagnosed a personality or character disorder and concentrated in therapy on self-defeating personality traits and defense mechanisms rather than mood. (Cognitive therapy is the only exception.) Today, subclinical depression is recognized as a disorder that can be responsive to medication. Therefore, many psychiatrists treating these patients now use Prozac along with psychotherapy or instead of it if the therapy alone has not worked.

• 3 •

Taking Prozac: The Basics

What causes depression?

The modern theory of depression hypothesizes that mood disorders are caused by imbalance in the number of small amino acid molecules, called neurotransmitters, that travel between nerves across the so-called synapses in the brain. Synapses are the spaces between two successive nerve fibers.

According to this theory, known as the biogenic amine hypothesis, the three major neurotransmitters located in brain synapses are: norepinephrine (NE), serotonin (SE), and dopamine (DA). The regulating mechanism is a complex one. It includes a process called uptake, whereby some of the neurotransmitter molecules in the synapse are absorbed back into the original nerve endings, where they either degenerate or are repackaged and sent back out again. Sometimes, as a result of genetic and environmental factors, this process produces imbalances in the amount of neurotransmitters in the synapses. An excess of one or more of the neurotransmitters is thought to lead to mania. A deficiency is thought to result in depression.

How do Prozac and other antidepressants work?

Prozac works by specifically inhibiting the uptake of serotonin at the nerve endings in the brain. This results in an increased concentration of serotonin at the synapse, which in turn increases the availability of serotonin at the critically important brain receptor sites, thought to result in normal nervous system transmission.

Prozac and the other SSRIs are highly specific in blocking the uptake only of serotonin, and not other neurotransmitters; that is why they are known as selective serotonin reuptake inhibitors (SSRIs). Because abnormalities in serotonin function have also been reported in obsessive-compulsive disorder, panic disorder, alcoholism, obesity, and other conditions, it is not surprising that some of these disorders have been successfully treated with Prozac and other SSRIs.

Tricyclic antidepressants, or TCAs, the most frequently used antidepressants over the past three or four decades prior to Prozac, were thought to alleviate depression by blocking norepinephrine and some serotonin uptake at the nerve terminals in the brain. This increased the levels of both neurotransmitters, permitting a return of normal nerve impulse flow, associated with the relief of depressive symptoms.

Other less commonly used older drugs, called MAOIs, or monoamine oxidase inhibitors, work in another way, by blocking the degradation of the enzyme monoamine oxidase at the nerve terminals. This leads to higher levels of norepinephrine and serotonin at the synapses and at critically important receptor sites. The final effects are similar to those achieved with the TCAs.

Prozac and other SSRIs including Zoloft, Paxil, Luvox, and Serzone, specifically block serotonin only.

How is Prozac usually given?

Most psychopharmacologists start patients on small doses of Prozac, anywhere from 10 to 20 mg per day. If a patient has not responded after two to four weeks, dosage may be increased to 40 mg and eventually even as much as 80 mg a day. Patients must be closely monitored on a weekly basis by a depression expert or psychopharmacologist who knows when to increase the drug and when to decrease or discontinue it if side effects become too disturbing.

How soon does a depressed mood begin to lift on Prozac?

Although a number of studies have shown that the depressed mood may begin to lift in a week, it generally takes at least two to three weeks for the patient and family to notice a real difference. The low mood may continue to lift for five to eight weeks before leveling off. In 65% to 70% of cases, the depression recedes within four to eight weeks. A patient should take a full dose of Prozac, under the supervision of an expert physician, for at least six weeks before concluding that the drug has failed to act on the depressive illness.

Occasionally people may claim to experience immediate relief. Although psychiatrists generally say this is the placebo effect, no psychopharmacologist can rule out the possibility that a given patient's metabolism may in rare instances react to the drug immediately, causing rapid changes in mood and behavior within one or two days. Occasionally, I find this instant response to be the case in patients who were previously hypomanic. A history of the way this patient and family members previously responded to this or other drugs often helps clarify whether this is the right antidepressant to take.

How long should I take Prozac?

Many psychopharmacologists suggest that Prozac (or any other antidepressant) be continued for three or four months after a single initial episode of depression has been alleviated. A smaller number of expert psychopharmacologists believe that the medicine should be continued as long as six to eight months.

In the case of recurrent unipolar depression, Prozac should be continued indefinitely to prevent future depressive episodes, if episodes occur yearly.

Similarly, patients who have suffered from bipolar manic depression (lithium treated) must be continued on Prozac for longer periods of time. In these instances, Prozac plus lithium may be used in the acute depressive phase, in the subsequent continuation phase for several months, and finally in the maintenance or prophylactic phase, often for years or a lifetime, to prevent future depressions from breaking through, if lithium alone does not prevent future depressions as well as future manic episodes.

With Prozac, I feel better than I have ever felt in my life. Will I ever be able to stop taking it, and if I do, what are the consequences?

One can stop taking Prozac at any time without concern for serious withdrawal effects due to the pharmacology of the drug itself. There are no symptoms of tolerance to Prozac or withdrawal symptoms of the sort that characterize drugs of abuse, including minor tranquilizers, sleeping pills, alcohol, and most illegal drugs.

However, patients who discontinue the drug will most often rebound into the previous depressive condition. Chronic diseases such as depression, obsessive-compulsive disorder, and bulimia are likely to return because most of these conditions are psychobiological. Once the treatment is removed, the biological component of the illness will revert to its original state, and the illness usually returns.

If the illness is intermittent and the patient goes off Prozac, the depression may not come back immediately, but it is very likely to return at some point in the future. After an initial episode of depression, the chances of experiencing a second episode are probably better than 50%. (A study in Europe found that the likelihood was much higher—between 70% and 80%.) Even more impressively, a second episode is followed by a third episode in 80% to 90% of the cases.

Does Prozac affect men differently from women? Young people differently from old people?

Prozac does not affect men differently from women or young people differently from older people. Younger healthy people, in general, take a stronger dose of Prozac than older people, those who are medically ill, or infirmed geriatric patients with depression. Children and young adolescents generally need smaller doses, but this is not well studied to date.

If someone I love is doing well on Prozac, but suddenly (or little by little) seems to be sliding back into depression, should I say something to the doctor? Will a stronger dose get the patient back to the previous level?

Usually, what is going on in such an instance is that the patient, after coming out of depression on

Prozac, forgets to take the medication or cuts down on the drug without the physician's knowledge. Sometimes the doctor and not the patient is to blame: a frequent reason for slipping back into depression after an excellent response is that the physician, typically someone who has not had extensive training and experience with Prozac and other antidepressant drugs, takes the patient off the drug too soon.

If these possibilities are eliminated and the patient is still losing ground, the dosage should be increased. The problem may be that although the dosage brought the patient out of the initial depression, the level of the drug in the blood did not remain high enough to prevent relapse.

The first time I took Prozac, I had a horrible time. The second time it went well. Why?

This phenomenon is not easily explicable but occurs with many medications, both in psychiatry and in general medicine. It is not uncommon to hear that a patient's first experience with an antidepressant drug was not successful but that the second time it went extremely well.

One possible explanation of this is the so-called placebo effect, present in 10% to 15% of patients. The placebo effect is usually thought of as influencing patients in a positive way: that is, their positive expectations or belief in the doctor may cause them to see immediate improvements even before the drug theoretically is supposed to work. But the placebo effect has a negative side also, for if the patient is worried or even phobic about taking a given drug, the anxiety can produce side effects for which the drug itself is not responsible, and these negative expectations may cause the patient to discontinue the medication prematurely, before it has had a chance to work. A related issue has to do with the patient's overall confidence in authorities, in this instance a physician. The more the patient trusts the doctor, the better the reaction to the drug is likely to be.

A second possible explanation has to do with the patient's metabolism, which may from time to time vary in its fluid and electrolyte balance, either as a result of taking other medications or of changing diet or fluid intake. Or the patient's metabolism may have simply changed in some way that at first glance is not easily understood by either the patient or the physician.

Finally, the patient may have been given too much of the drug on the first occasion. On the second try, if the drug is given in a much smaller amount, with the dosage being raised gradually, the results may be highly effective, and rewarding.

Does Prozac lose its effectiveness after continued usage?

No, it does not. Once Prozac has sufficient time to build up in the body and relieve the symptoms of depression, the patient takes either the same dosage or less during both the continuation phase, which lasts two to three months, and later during the long-term maintenance phase.

What happens if the dosage is lowered?

About four to six months after the depression has been alleviated, and assuming the symptoms have not returned, the decision could be made to lower the dosage. If the depression does not return, fine. However, if the patient slides back into depression on the lower dose, it is better to restore the full amount as a maintenance dose. In many patients with recurrent unipolar depression, the smaller dose will protect the patient from immediate relapse, but in some the smaller dose is insufficient and future recurrent depressions eventually reemerge. This simply tells the physician and the patient that the maintenance dose needs to be kept at a higher level, often the same level required to alleviate the acute depressive episode. This general principle is also true for lithium and other antidepressant drugs.

In my clinical experience with thousands of depressed patients, a certain number, year after year, come to the office in a depression, take an antidepressant, and then once the depression is alleviated, stop their office visits and go off the drug on their own. In these instances, after a relapse, the antidepressant usually has to be reintroduced at the previous therapeutic level or at an even higher level before the depression again disappears.

Is Prozac habit-forming or addictive?

There is no evidence in laboratory studies of Prozac in animals or in clinical studies with thousands of patients that it is either habit-forming or addictive. The two common properties of addictive substances are tolerance (the need to take increasingly stronger doses to achieve the same result) and withdrawal (the collection of disturbing psychic and psychological symptoms that occur when an addictive substance is removed from a patient's system). Patients who do well on 20 mg of Prozac for long periods of time do not become tolerant and therefore need 30 or 40 mg to obtain the same result. Likewise, when patients go off Prozac, there are no moderate to severe withdrawal symptoms such as diarrhea, anxiety, pains, nasal stuffiness, and insomnia. These symptoms may be seen in addicted patients when they withdraw from habit-forming tranquilizers such as Xanax, Ativan, Klonopin, Librium, Miltown, and all of the typical sleeping medications, including barbiturates, Halcion, Restoril, Dalmane, and chloral hydrate.

What is the difference between Prozac in liquid and capsule or pill form?

In terms of antidepressant effects, there are no differences. The main difference is that the liquid form makes it possible to take a much smaller dose with the use of an ordinary dropper and a set of kitchen measuring spoons. With the liquid, one can take 20 mg in a teaspoon, 10 mg in a half teaspoon, 5 mg in a quarter of a teaspoon, or even, theoretically, 2.5 mg in an eighth of a teaspoon, which the pharmacy translates into a specific number of drops. The smallest dose of Prozac in capsule form is 10 mg. At the present time Prozac is unavailable in pill or tablet form.

What percentage of patients take Prozac for disorders other than depression?

Approximately a third. This percentage is gaining steadily with the recent publicity about Prozac's effectiveness in treating patients with nondepressive disorders, including obsessive-compulsive disorder, bulimia, and personality disorders.

What is the usual dosage of Prozac?

The standard dose is 20 mg of Prozac a day and 5 to 10 mg for children and the elderly. Dosage must be individualized.

What is the lowest dose shown to be effective, and when is this indicated?

Anecdotal reports by individual psychiatrists suggest that the lowest dose that seems to have been effective is 2.5 to 5 mg a day. As noted above, this may be indicated in young children, some very elderly patients, and patients who develop side effects on a standard dose.

What is the highest safe dosage of Prozac, and when is this indicated?

Individuals differ, both in their genetic tolerance for a given dose and in the side effects they experience, but in general, the maximum recommended dose is 80 mg a day.

However, that dosage has been exceeded occasionally with very overweight patients. Some obese patients have come out of depressive episodes after being given over 80 mg in select cases where safety has been maintained. Such a dosage is not advised in general because there are potential safety concerns in patients taking over 80 mg a day.

What time of the day is Prozac usually taken?

Prozac is usually taken in the morning after breakfast, which seems to produce fewer side effects, particularly nausea and insomnia. But some patients have been able to tolerate it with other meals or at other times of the day, including bedtime, without adverse side effects. Many patients take Prozac at a time when it is most convenient for them or simply easy to remember, whether in the morning, after dinner, or at bedtime. *(See Chapter 4: Side Effects.)*

Can you overdose on Prozac?

Not easily. During preclinical trials with Prozac up to 1993, no deaths occurred in patients receiving Prozac in normal doses. Two deaths were reported during comparative clinical trials, but in both cases other drugs were involved, so the role of Prozac is not clear. Another thirty-two patients recovered after overdose without any lasting harm, including one who reportedly took 3000 mg of Prozac, which is over thirty-seven times the recommended maximum dose of 80 mg.

In contrast, it is easy to overdose with other antidepressants such as the TCAs and MAOIs due to the toxic effects of high doses on the heart. With Prozac, even in large amounts, the risk of serious cardiovascular or neurologic harm is very small. Prozac should be considered one of the safest of all the antidepressant drugs.

If my spouse is taking Prozac and I take a capsule by mistake, will it hurt me?

No. A single dose of Prozac should not hurt a healthy person. The possible side effects and risks of using Prozac in small doses in conjunction with tricyclic and tetracyclic antidepressants appear to be minimal.

However, the use of Prozac with MAOI antidepressants such as Nardil, Parnate or Marplan is considered dangerous. Prozac taken by mistake with an MAOI could conceivably cause a toxic reaction with elevated blood pressure, nausea, vomiting, or shock. Immediate transport to an emergency ward is indicated if such symptoms follow. A patient switching from an MAOI to Prozac must wait at least two weeks. A patient switching from Prozac to an MAOI must wait at least *five* weeks. Failure to observe these precautions can result in severe toxic reactions and even death. *(See Chapter 7 for more information on MAOIs.)*

Is Prozac a drug that has to be taken forever?

It depends on the individual. The evidence suggests that between 20% and 30% of patients have only a single depression in their lives. Four to six months after their depression has lifted, these patients can taper off Prozac without recurrence and may never have to take Prozac or another antidepressant again.

However, millions of people suffer from recurrent depression. These people are much better off taking Prozac or another antidepressant on a permanent basis to prevent future attacks. This is also true for those manic-depressive patients who are on lithium but who nonetheless find that the depressive phase still breaks through. For these people, lithium and Prozac or another antidepressant have to be taken together on a long-term basis.

Keep in mind, though, that older antidepressants have been around for thirty to thirty-five years. Although some patients have been successfully taking Prozac for as long as seven or eight years, Prozac is still essentially a new drug, and we simply do not know its long-term effects. There is still reason for caution.

How does my doctor know how much Prozac I should be taking? Do I have to take periodic blood tests so that the doctor can monitor the level of Prozac in my system? Or is it just the way I feel?

Because studies have not correlated a specific blood level of Prozac with therapeutic results, blood tests are not routinely taken. This is in direct contrast to some other antidepressants. For instance, with at least four tricyclic antidepressants (imipramine, desipramine, nortriptyline, and amitriptyline), blood levels may be routinely taken by some psychiatrists, including myself, because certain levels are needed to achieve a therapeutic window effect, and hence the blood test serves as a guide to the psychiatrist as to the dosage required.

With Prozac, on the other hand, the appropriate dosage, for the most part, corresponds simply to weight and age. Patients of average age and weight (for men that is 150 pounds, mean age 35; for women that is 120 pounds, mean age 35) need approximately 20 mg of Prozac a day, with the very young and very old taking smaller doses. But the average dose is not necessarily the correct one for a given individual. Ultimately, the way a patient feels is the most important determinant of the final dosage, along with the patient's specific metabolism and genetic factors.

Is it easy to withdraw from Prozac?

Yes. If necessary, patients taking doses between 5 and 20 mg can stop taking the medication immediately. However, as a general rule in medicine, it is always better to taper off drugs. Patients taking higher doses can taper off over a week to ten days by taking smaller doses every other day and then every third day before discontinuing. Prozac's metabolism would suggest that coming off the medication should not be of concern due to the long half-life of the antidepressant, which means it is tapering off slowly by itself after it has been discontinued.

When is Prozac contraindicated?

Patients who have severe kidney or liver disease should generally not take Prozac because it is metabolized in the liver and excreted in the kidneys. A specialist in kidney or liver disease should be consulted. With severe impairment of either or both of these organs, Prozac can build up in the blood to a very high, possibly dangerous, level. Prozac is also contraindicated in patients with severe allergies and in patients who break out in a rash or hives after starting Prozac treatment.

Is Prozac available in foreign countries?

Patients taking Prozac outside the United States should have a signed note from their American physician explaining what the medication is and what it is being used for, as required by customs. Prozac is available in many countries under foreign trade names. If the term "Prozac" is not used in a given country, the generic name fluoxetine should be used instead.

If the patient talks to a pharmacy or physician ahead of time, a courier package of Prozac can be delivered within twenty-four to seventy-two hours to most major cities of the world.

There is no need to be unduly concerned about hot weather, mild dehydration, or skipping an occasional meal (as one should be with lithium), none of which should cause any unusual symptoms with Prozac. However, normal food, fluid, and salt intake are required and should be maintained.

What about alcohol and Prozac?

A general medical principle is that even nonalcoholics should drink only moderately or not at all while taking any medications, including Prozac. After being stabilized on Prozac or other antidepressants, patients who do not have an alcohol problem are permitted to have a glass of wine at dinner, provided that no adverse effects on judgment or mood take place. Obviously, patients who are taking Prozac or any other psychotropic drugs should not use alcohol prior to driving. Most medical authorities argue that no alcohol should be used by anyone who plans to drive.

If the patient is alcoholic, as is often the case with those suffering from major depression, dysthymia, and bipolar manic depression (due to a genetic alcoholic predisposition), it is imperative to abstain from alcohol completely.

Interestingly, a least one study suggests that a dosage of 60 mg of Prozac may cause heavy drinkers to drink less alcohol but not to smoke fewer cigarettes.

Will Prozac make me more or less hungry?

In many patients, Prozac causes mild nausea during the first few days of treatment. In addition, as a result of the biochemical effects of Prozac on carbohydrate craving and overall metabolism, many—but not all—patients feel less hungry than they did before taking the drug. Most patients either maintain their weight or lose a few pounds—in stark contrast to the older antidepressants, which frequently cause weight gain.

Is dieting allowed when receiving Prozac treatment?

A sensible diet, with moderate caloric restriction, should present no problem for someone taking Prozac, especially if supervised by the psychopharmacologist in conjunction with either a nutritionist or a diet program approved by the American Medical Association. In general, stay away from inappropriate crash diets or fad programs.

What is the role of the family of a patient taking Prozac?

The family of a patient on Prozac should familiarize itself with the nature of the depression and be particularly on guard if there is a past, present, or family history of suicide ideation, negative reactions to specific antidepressants, or mania exists. Probably the most important step they can take is to understand that depression is a psychobiologic illness. The patient is not responsible for the depression and cannot simply "buck up."

Furthermore, the family should consult with the doctor and read as much material as possible in order to understand the purpose, effects, and side effects of Prozac and other psychopharmacologic agents. This is especially true when the patient is a young adolescent or an elderly person who is dependent on the family for keeping regular appointments with the psychopharmacologist and sometimes with a second therapist, whom I also recommend for about a third of my depressed patients on antidepressants. The family members need to understand that these repeated visits serve an important monitoring function of the patient's clinical state, side effects, and general blood chemistries.

How long does Prozac last in the body?

One way of answering this question is to look at the half-life. The pharmacologic term "half-life" is used to describe the time it takes for the drug in the blood to decrease by half of its original administered amount. The half-life of Prozac is approximately one to three days, while the half-life of its breakdown metabolic product (metabolite), norfluoxetine, ranges from seven to fifteen days, meaning that Prozac and its metabolite leave the system gradually. In comparison with other antidepressants, including the SSRIs Paxil and Zoloft, the half-life of Prozac is extended. The half-life of Zoloft is about twenty-six hours and that of Paxil about twenty-one hours.

The extended half-life of Prozac may have several advantages. First of all, upon discontinuation it is less likely to precipitate withdrawal symptoms than an antidepressant with a short half-life. Within only twelve hours after suddenly discontinuing a large dose of a tricyclic antidepressant or an MAOI medication, a patient may experience nausea, dizziness, vomiting, sleep disturbance, symptoms of rapid withdrawal, and even rebound hypomania or mania in bipolar depressions not simultaneously treated with lithium. Prozac's extended half-life prevents these acute withdrawal symptoms.

The stable blood levels associated with an extended half-life may help prevent relapse when the dose is lowered or when the patient simply forgets to take the medication for a day or two.

Will Prozac help me sleep better at night?

If Prozac successfully alleviates major depression and dysthymia, sleep usually improves as well, since insomnia is a characteristic symptom of these illnesses.

On the other hand, in the beginning, Prozac does have the side effect of causing mild insomnia. Patients usually complain about this the first few days after starting the drug. As the symptoms of major depression begin to recede, however, this side effect usually disappears and normal sleep is restored.

Does Prozac affect the thought processes? Does it cause dullness of mind?

Reports in the scientific literature do not indicate that Prozac adversely affects thinking or cognitive processes such as memory and recall, and patients have not complained to me that they have experienced a dull feeling mentally after taking Prozac. On the other hand, once the depression lifts, patients feel sharper. In contrast, patients on high doses of tricyclics and MAOIs frequently complain of problems with memory and trouble finding words at the end of a sentence.

• 4 •

Side Effects

In the past, patients taking the tried and true older antidepressants found that while their depression would often lift, the dry mouth, constipation, dizziness, weight gain, and rapid heartbeat (to name only a few common side effects) were uncomfortable and disturbing. Many times these side effects led patients to discontinue the medication on their own. With Prozac, most of these problems have been eliminated. My patients make comments such as these: "After going off my old antidepressant and starting on Prozac, I can't believe the difference. I used to have such a dry mouth. No more! And to have this happen in three or four weeks, I can't believe it. I feel absolutely back to my normal self."

At the same time, Prozac, like every other drug, does have side effects, most of which are extremely minor—especially when compared to the bleak despondency that caused these people to show up in my office.

But some patients—far fewer than with the earlier antidepressant medications—find the side effects difficult to tolerate. This chapter focuses on these reactions, from the fleeting few days of nausea and sleeplessness that Prozac may cause in the beginning of treatment to the surprising (and, for many patients, wonderful) weight loss that may also accompany treatment.

What are the main side effects of Prozac?

Let me reiterate: after numerous clinical trials, it is apparent that, compared with other older antidepressants, Prozac has an exceptionally low incidence of side effects. Nevertheless, there are *some* side effects. In clinical trials of about three thousand patients, the following reactions were seen:

- Nausea. Some 21% of the patients in clinical trials complained about nausea, making it the most frequent side effect associated with Prozac. However, only 2% of the patients actually vomited. Complaints of nausea were most frequent during the first few days to two weeks, after which the number of complaints dropped precipitously. After a few weeks, almost all of the nausea subsided. Nausea is Prozac's most notable side effect, so it is worth pointing out that in clinical studies comparing Prozac with tricyclic antidepressants and a placebo, 15% of those taking the TCAs also complained of nausea, and so did 10% of those receiving a placebo.

- Headaches. About 20% of the Prozac patients experienced this side effect, but it caused only 2% to stop taking the drug. Again, approximately equal numbers of those taking the TCA imipramine or placebo also complained about headache.

- Nervousness and anxiety. Between 10% and 15% of the Prozac patients registered these complaints. For the most part, these side effects were relatively mild, causing only 5% of the patients actually to discontinue treatment.

- Insomnia. About 14% of the patients had difficulty sleeping, and 2% discontinued the drug as a result.

- Drowsiness. About 12% of the patients were bothered by drowsiness.

- Anorexia. This affected 9% of the patients. Some investigators (but not most) have concluded that this could explain why most Prozac patients fail to gain weight, in contrast to patients who take most of the tricyclic and MAOI antidepressants. This is one incredibly important aspect of Prozac that makes it particularly desirable among patients who are obese or tend to gain weight easily, especially with other antidepressant drugs.

- Diarrhea. About 12% of the patients experienced diarrhea.

- Dry mouth. Only 9.5% of Prozac patients experienced dry mouth—a stunning improvement over the 64.3% of patients taking tricyclic antidepressants who complained about this irritating (for some) symptom. Sucking hard candy helps.

- Sweating and tremor. These symptoms affected about 8% of the patients taking Prozac.

- Rash. Rashes showed up in about 3% of the patients, a figure not so different from the 4% who break out in rashes after taking tricyclic antidepressants (and the 2% of patients taking a placebo who develop a rash). Typically, the rash appeared during the first few weeks and usually disappeared within a week, whether or not the patient stopped taking Prozac. Occasionally, hives, pains in the joints, or other systemic problems occurred simultaneously with the rash. For this reason, most physicians recommend that, if a rash appears, the patient should immediately stop taking the medication.

Laboratory data have shown no evidence of damage to the liver, kidneys, bone marrow, or heart associated with Prozac.

What other less common side effects are reported with Prozac?

As with every drug in existence, the list of less common side effects is long and extends into virtually every system in the body. At least 1% of the patients on Prozac have complained on at least one occasion of chills, disturbed dreams, bronchitis, agitation, or excessive yawning.

Other side effects experienced by at least one patient in a thousand include, among many other reactions, feeling hung over, jaw pain, neck pain, excessive belching, gingivitis, thirst, hypothyroidism, anemia, weight gain (a larger number of patients lose weight), arthritis, bursitis, acne, loss of hair, conjunctivitis, ear pain, eye pain, and various urinary disturbances.

Infrequent cardiovascular side effects include angina pectoris, arrhythmia, hypertension, hypotension, and migraine headaches.

Infrequent nervous system reactions include abnormal gait, amnesia, apathy, convulsions, hallucinations, hostility, and paranoia.

Then there are the "rare" side effects, which occur in fewer than one person in a thousand. These extremely unusual events include enlarged abdomen, thrombophlebitis, colitis, duodenal ulcer, increased salivation, hepatitis, jaundice, stomach ulcer, goiter, hyperthyroidism, dehydration, gout, osteoporosis, rheumatoid arthritis, antisocial reaction, eczema, unwanted hair growth, psoriasis, and many other side effects too numerous (and uncommon) to name here.

The important point is that compared to the older classically used antidepressants, the side effects of Prozac are infrequent and mild—even in overdose. Most of the older antidepressants have similarly long lists of side effects, most of which are rare, although they are listed in the *Physicians' Desk Reference* and the package inserts, often to protect the manufacturer as well as the patient.

Why do some patients who take Prozac discontinue treatment?

Many patients who stop taking Prozac on their own do so because they find the side effects of slight nausea and insomnia unbearable or are too impatient to wait for early side effects to recede. Patients who are prone to hysterical reactions or those who are phobic about taking pills are often doomed to discontinue Prozac or any other medication from the outset.

The main complaints that cause patients to discontinue treatment are, in order of frequency, nausea, nervousness, insomnia, anxiety, tremor, headache, drowsiness, diarrhea, dizziness, sweating, and dry mouth.

The numbers and percentages for each of these categories are small. Nausea, the most common adverse reaction associated with stopping treatment, caused between 3% and 4% of the people tested to stop taking the drug. Nervousness and insomnia influenced another 2% to 3% to discontinue treatment. Not one of the other side effects involved in ending treatment affected more than 2% of those tested.

Does Prozac cause waking in the night?

About 14% of patients taking Prozac experience some insomnia, especially in the beginning of treatment. Fot that reason, most patients take Prozac in the morning. (A much smaller number of patients find Prozac to be sedating; for them, it is better to take the medicine at night.) It does not cause waking throughout the night or in the early morning.

Does Prozac cause nightmares?

It is highly unlikely that Prozac causes nightmares, since, like other antidepressants, it suppresses rapid eye movement (REM) sleep, which is when most nightmares take place. However, as with all antidepressants, some patients on Prozac do report nightmares, and a small percentage of patients have reported abnormal dreams.

What is the total percentage of patients who stop taking Prozac because of the side effects?

In clinical trials, 17% of those taking Prozac discontinued treatment, compared to a full 31% of those taking the tricyclic antidepressants.

Does the size of the dose determine the side effects?

The incidence of most side effects, including nausea, anxiety, anorexia, diarrhea, insomnia, tremor, and drowsiness, increases with the size of the dose.

Will Prozac make my hypomanic or manic highs feel better or worse? I am a little high most of the time. What will Prozac do to me?

Prozac is really contraindicated in cases in which the patient has been experiencing the manic or hypomanic ups that are the most important signs and symptoms of manic-depressive illness or other bipolar disorders. With or without the depressed downs, patients with a history of clear-cut hypomanic or manic episodes should not be treated solely with Prozac or other antidepressants because these drugs can induce a full-blown manic or even psychotic episode. (The same problem may exist when a patient is diagnosed with major depressive disorder but the family history shows strong signs of bipolar disorder.)

However, Prozac can be an important part of a coordinated treatment program when combined with lithium or the alternatives Tegretol or Depakote. If the mood swings have been treated with these medications and as a result, the highs have been stabilized but the lows have not, the addition of small amounts of Prozac may help stabilize the overall manic-depressive condition.

In my experience, patients with hypomania or mania should under no circumstances take Prozac or any other antidepressant drug without first being stabilized on lithium or one of its alternatives. If such a mistake is made by the physician, the patient may report feeling supertransformed in what is becoming a manic psychosis that will require hospitalization.

Needless to say, if the Prozac patient on or off lithium is having this reaction, the immediate discontinuation of Prozac, an increase in lithium, and possible hospitalization are required.

However, caution must be taken when combining Prozac with antimanic drugs. In three isolated instances, the so-called toxic serotonin syndrome has been reported in patients taking a combination of Prozac and Tegretol, and in one case—the only one in eight years—it appeared in a patient taking Prozac and lithium. The symptoms of the serotonin syndrome are serious and best treated in a hospital. They include shivering, tremor, increased diarrhea, dizziness, loss of coordination, and involuntary muscle movements.

What would be the consequences in a very suicidal patient who becomes anxious after being given Prozac?

In about 10% to 15% of depressed patients, anxiety increases after taking Prozac, especially during the first two to three weeks. This effect gradually diminishes, and most patients can cope with the change.

But with highly suicidal patients, this slight increase in anxiety could conceivably push them over the edge. For that reason, suicidal patients should be monitored closely as they begin to emerge from their depressions. This is true with Prozac—and equally true with every other antidepressant on the market.

How valid are the claims that Prozac may induce weight loss?

In thousands of patients studied in clinical trials before December 1987, Prozac was repeatedly found to induce weight loss, making it the first antidepressant ever marketed in the United States for which this is true. One study found that after six weeks, patients taking the older, tricyclic antidepressants gained about one pound while those on Prozac lost weight. And the heavier they were, the more they lost. Patients of normal weight lost about two pounds, while those considered obese dropped an average of seven pounds in six weeks. (After long-term treatment, the weight loss reached a plateau.) Other clinical trials show that after six weeks, patients of normal weight lost two to four pounds, while those who were overweight dropped an average of four pounds. In addition, about 13% of the

patients in a controlled clinical trial lost more than
5% of their body weight while taking Prozac.

The explanation for the weight loss is simple: the
patients ate less while on Prozac. But why they ate
less is not agreed upon.

Although the weight loss Prozac produces is not
enormous, it is statistically significant. Psychologi-
cally, the weight loss can be even more important.
Many patients, especially women, are devastated
when one of the older and well-known antidepressants causes their dress size to grow as their depression diminishes. Prozac, to the delight of most, has
an opposite effect.

On the other hand, a small percentage of patients
paradoxically gain weight, although this happens far
less often than has been seen with tricyclic antidepressants, MAOI antidepressants, lithium, Depakote,
and Tegretol, all of which are associated with some
degree of weight gain in one-third of patients taking
these medications.

Can obesity be treated with Prozac?

Clinical trials using Prozac in obese patients who
are not depressed are still ongoing. Results are
promising, but the FDA has not yet decided to allow
Prozac to be marketed as a specific treatment for
weight loss.

Can bulimia be treated with Prozac?

Between 1.3% and 10.1% of all American women
suffer from bulimia nervosa, a serious, sometimes
even fatal syndrome that causes them to attempt to
control their weight by alternating binges of compulsive eating with vomiting and laxative abuse. A
study of 387 bulimic women divided them into three
equal groups. One group was given 20 mg of Prozac
a day, one group was given a daily dose of 60 mg,

and one group received a placebo. The results were encouraging. By the end of the eight-week trial, the women on Prozac reported fewer eating binges and less vomiting than the women who had been given a placebo. (Reductions also emerged in depression and carbohydrate craving, among other eating-related measurements.) In addition, those taking the larger dose of Prozac were more successful at changing their behavior than those on the smaller doses.

Although the participants who received Prozac reported a higher incidence of insomnia, nausea, and other side effects, they did not drop out of the program at a greater rate than those on the placebo, suggesting once more that the side effects of Prozac are relatively tolerable.

Can Prozac make me irritable or angry?

It depends on your basic temperament and chemistry. Patients who begin taking Prozac when they are both deeply depressed and highly irritable usually find that irritability diminishes or disappears along with the depression. This has the effect of improving their relationships with their spouses, peers, colleagues, and children. Spouses and grown children sitting in my office with their formerly depressed loved ones have often told me how much easier it is to get along now that the crankiness or anger outbursts have faded along with the depression. Of course, many depressed patients are withdrawn rather than angry.

It is another story with patients who have a tendency toward bipolar mood swings with manic highs characterized by irritability, anger, and paranoid delusions rather than by euphoria and grandiosity. If they take Prozac during a depressed phase and have not been previously stabilized on lithium, the hypomanic or manic side of the mood may emerge in the form of these symptoms.

How can restlessness and irritability that I felt when taking Prozac be reduced?

A lower dosage may help. Although most patients take 10 or 20 mg a day of Prozac, as little as 2.5 mg a day may be effective in some patients who are sensitive to the usual recommended dose.

Can Prozac make me complacent?

There is no report of Prozac causing complacency in any patients, although drowsiness, a side effect in about 12% of patients, might be misinterpreted by some as complacency. Complacency can be a symptom of a depressive personality (dysthymia), subclinical depression, the down side of cyclothymia, or a major depression itself.

Will Prozac affect my sexuality?

It may. Although early studies indicated that the incidence of sexual side effects associated with antidepressants was quite low, recent studies suggest otherwise. About 25% to 35% of patients taking all antidepressants, including Prozac, seem to have some sexual side effects including *decreased* desire, potency problems, delayed ejaculation, and trouble reaching orgasm.

Nonetheless, although a number of patients do report some altered sexual functioning with Prozac, and also with the newer SSRIs, they seldom stop taking the drug for this reason. Although they're not pleased to have sexual difficulties, they are so grateful to feel normal in other respects that usually they learn to cope.

Other people (including three elderly men who reportedly had sexual functioning restored after many years of dysfunction) experience no problems in sexual functioning and often find themselves more interested in sex than they had been. Since depression causes a decrease in libido, most patients who recover from depression can confidently expect an *increase* in sexual desire. By lifting the depression, Prozac increases the libido and makes it easier to find enjoyment in all kinds of activities, including sex. However, the price may be delayed orgasm in one third of both men and women.

According to at least one non-scientifically controlled study published on six men and women receiving SSRIs and experiencing the typical sexual side effects, most of these symptoms were improved with the administration of Yohimbine.

Why do different antidepressants produce different side effects?

Different antidepressants have varied side effects because they act differently in the central nervous system. Specifically, the side effects depend on how the medication interacts with the neurotransmitters released at the nerve synapse and with the receptors located on the nerve cell on the other side of the synaptic gap. Prozac and the other SSRI classical drugs including setraline (Zoloft) and paroxetine (Paxil) selectively make certain that the neurotransmitter serotonin is not reabsorbed into the nerve, thus causing the brain serotonin levels to increase specifically. In contrast, and as I have already noted, older antidepressants block the uptake of the neurotransmitters norepinephrine and dopamine as well as serotonin. Effexor, the latest antidepressant to be FDA approved, increases both norepinephrine and serotonin levels, but has a mild side effect profile like the SSRIs.

Different mechanisms of action produce different

side effects. The blockage of norepinephrine uptake, for instance, can produce tachycardia, tremor, and sexual dysfunction. Blocking dopamine (a process important to the antidepressants Asendin and Wellbutrin) can produce movement disorders and changes in the endocrine system. Blocking serotonin avoids those problems for the most part but can create instead gastric distress, insomnia, and anxiety.

In addition, many antidepressants work on the other side of the synaptic gap, blocking the receptors that normally pick up the neurotransmitters. Again, the side effects depend on which receptors (among them $Alpha_1$, Dopamine D_2, Histamine H_1, and muscarinic receptors) are being blocked. Block the Histamine H_1 receptors and you're likely to see sedation and weight gain. Block the muscarinic receptors, and you can expect blurred vision, a dry mouth, constipation, and an impaired memory.

The more an antidepressant participates in these processes, the more side effects it is likely to produce. Thus, a tricyclic antidepressant such as amitriptyline (Elavil), which blocks the uptake of norepinephrine and serotonin as well as all four receptors listed above, is also associated with a much higher incidence of side effects than is Prozac, which is more limited, and thus more specific in its action.

Unlike older medications, Prozac blocks receptors only minimally, making it the first but not the only antidepressant for which this is true. Other SSRIs and Effexor also interfere very weakly with the receptors.

Why does Prozac sometimes produce a "revved up" feeling?

Since Prozac selectively blocks the uptake of serotonin, which specifically creates anxiety and gastrointestinal disturbances, anxiety is a common side effect (as is nausea). Especially in the beginning, a certain number of people also experience the related sensations of restlessness, nervousness, agitation, decreased appetite, and trouble sleeping. They simply can't sit still.

One of my patients, D.W., is a 35-year-old male diabetic with a history of major depression and some experience with other antidepressants. "I felt like I was racing all the time," he told me. "I couldn't relax. I couldn't sit down. I was nervous, uncomfortable and fidgety." Despite the initial speediness and discomfort, he felt that Prozac helped him feel "more up, more outgoing," and the revved up feeling was curbed by decreasing the dosage of Prozac after week one.

Although this feeling of being revved up is a real effect of Prozac and some of the SSRIs, a major study has shown these activating effects to be only slightly greater than the activating effects seen in depressed patients taking a standard comparison drug, imipramine (Tofranil). In clinical studies, patients who made the decision to stop taking either drug blamed it on these adverse activating effects in approximately equal numbers.

What are the most common sedating side effects of Prozac?

About 12% of patients taking Prozac (compared to about 24% of these treated with tricyclics) complain of drowsiness, and 4% have reported a feeling of asthenia, or weakness. If the feeling doesn't go away within a few days, a smaller dose of Prozac should be tried.

In addition, in placebo-controlled clinical trials, 4.2% of the 1730 patients taking Prozac complained of fatigue and 1.9% reported feelings of sedation.

Has Prozac been adequately tested for long-term side effects?

No, if you define long-term as I do, as being 25 to 30 years. Prozac has only been available since 1987. Most patients who have been on long-term Prozac since then have been on it for a maximum of five to seven years. Not until patients have been adequately observed and tested on Prozac for fifteen to thirty years can one say that the medication has been adequately tested for long-term side effects.

• 5 •

Prozac and the Body:
Physical Interactions

Depressed people are sometimes told to "buck up," snap out of it, quit whining, or get their act together. But it doesn't work that way. Major depression is a physiological condition, many varieties of which have been shown to be genetically inherited. It is characterized by disturbances of appetite, sex, sleep, and mood, all of which appear to have their primary location in an area of the brain called the hypothalamus, which acts as a control center for these physiological functions and needs and is influenced by other biochemical processes in the brain and the body. Major depression is not just a psychological reaction to some real or imaginary loss; it is biological with psychological components and effects.

The sole use of Prozac (and other antidepressants) depends in part on the patient's physical health. This chapter answers some important questions about the interaction of depression, antidepressants, and the human body.

How is Prozac absorbed, metabolized, and excreted in the body?

Prozac (fluoxetine) is easily absorbed after being swallowed, whether or not the patient has recently eaten. (However, the presence of food does slow down the process somewhat.) Once the medication is absorbed, it is metabolized primarily by the liver, which turns fluoxetine into its breakdown product (or metabolite), norfluoxetine. Both chemicals block the uptake of serotonin.

About a month after beginning treatment, the concentration of both fluoxetine and norfluoxetine reaches a stable level. Part of this stability derives from the fact that as an antidepressant Prozac has a long half-life, meaning that it takes a relatively long time to decrease by half its originally administered amount. The half-life of fluoxetine is one to three days, and the half-life of norfluoxetine ranges from seven to fifteen days–a long time compared to the other SSRIs on the market. Prozac lingers. An advantage to its long half-life is that patients who stop taking the drug, even abruptly, are unlikely to go through withdrawal, which often occurs with antidepressant drugs that have a shorter half-life. Similarly, a patient who forgets to take a pill for a day or two will not be plunged into despair as a result of the lapse.

On the other hand, sometimes you might not want Prozac to be in the body, perhaps because of a medical emergency that requires another drug. In switching to an MAOI, a patient has to wait up to five weeks, since the two drugs together can be lethal and are thus contraindicated. In that situation, the long half-life could conceivably be a disadvantage.

Prozac is excreted primarily through the kidney,

with about 80% of the drug eliminated by the urine and 15% by the feces.

Although more long-term studies need to be done, the process of absorption, metabolism, and excretion of Prozac seems to be the same in the elderly and in the young.

Can I take Prozac if I'm alcoholic and have liver disease?

Because Prozac is metabolized principally by the liver, depressed or alcoholic patients with liver disfunction should be given either a lower dose of Prozac (or any other SSRI antidepressant) or none at all. A liver that is already overtaxed will take significantly more time to metabolize the drug. Regular monitoring of liver funtioning is necessary. Researchers have discovered that patients with normal livers require no more than three days before the amount of Prozac in the body diminishes to one-half, while patients with cirrhosis of the liver need over a week—7.6 days—to reach the same point. In addition, the study found that Prozac's metabolite, norfluoxetine, also took several days longer to be flushed out of the system when liver disease was present.

What are the effects of Prozac on kidney function?

Because the kidneys are responsible for the elimination of Prozac, an impaired and hence less efficient kidney may cause the drug to accumulate in the body. For this reason, patients with renal disease, as evidenced by high BUN or serum creatinine, including those undergoing hemodialysis, should take smaller than normal doses of Prozac. (Again, the same recommendation holds for patients with kidney disease who are receiving other SSRIs for their depression. Regular monitoring is required and a nephrologist should be consulted.)

Does Prozac affect thyroid function?

Depressed patients who come to my office for a complete diagnostic evaluation are first required to have a complete physical exam, an EKG, and a blood chemistry profile that measures, among other substances, the level of thyroid hormone. Because an amount below the normal range is sufficient in itself in some cases to cause depression, patients with underactive thyroids may need first and foremost to take thyroid medication. If the depression has not begun to disappear on thyroid hormone alone after seven to ten days, a trial of an antidepressant is initiated. However, if patients are already in a major depression superimposed on hypothyroidism, they may need an antidepressant as well as the thyroid hormone.

Fortunately, studies have shown no important interactions between Prozac and thyroid hormone. The two medications can be taken simultaneously. Thyroid hormone is usually given as levothyroxin. Cytomel or T_3 (triiodothyronine) is given to boost the action of tricyclic antidepressants and used as a step-up treatment with Prozac if the antidepressant is not doing the job on its own.

To date, no clear-cut warning has been given regarding any important adverse effects of Prozac on the thyroid. Very infrequent cases of hypothyroidism have been reported with patients on Prozac. Even more rarely, goiter and hyperthyroidism have been reported, although they probably are not related to the Prozac treatment.

What are the effects of Prozac on the heart?

The effect of Prozac on the normal heart is minimal. A study of 312 patients revealed no clinically significant changes in the electrocardiogram. Unlike many older antidepressants, Prozac does not cause the heart to beat more quickly in the vast majority of patients. Indeed, researchers have found exactly the opposite: the pulse rate of patients on Prozac actually slows down by about three beats a minute.

However, general caution should be exercised with patients who have high blood pressure or other heart disorders. The dosage of the drug should be watched carefully on initiation and in many cases decreased to 10 mg per day, where the patient would otherwise begin at 20 mg daily.

How does Prozac compare to other antidepressants for patients with heart disease?

For patients with heart disease, Prozac is one of the safest antidepressants on the market. Patients taking tricyclics and MAOI antidepressants are at a higher risk of cardiac complications than patients taking any of the SSRIs such as Prozac, Paxil, and Zoloft, as well as Wellbutrin and Effexor.

Will Prozac affect my cholesterol count?

Cholesterol count does not seem to be related to Prozac intake.

Is the central nervous system in any way affected adversely by Prozac?

Prozac is remarkably benign, all in all. But as with any drug, there are the rare exceptions. For instance, twelve patients out of six thousand studied had seizures—a rate similar to that of most other antidepressants. Infrequently, there have been reports of abnormal gait, apathy, central nervous system stimulation, delusions, depersonalization, along with dysphoria, hallucinations, hostility, incoordination, paranoia, and other reactions. In very rare cases, an abnormal electroencephalogram has been reported. As with all the antidepressants, there are other highly unusual side effects as well.

But it is reassuring to note that the worst of these reactions occurs in fewer than one patient out of a hundred (and often fewer than one patient in a thousand). The most common adverse effects on the central nervous system, reported in more than 1% of the patients, are abnormal dreams and agitation.

Is Prozac helpful in the commonly manifested depressed mood seen in Parkinson's disease?

To date, the evidence is not encouraging. There have been reports of increased motor disability in four patients with Parkinson's disease who have been exposed to Prozac.

Is Prozac helpful in the commonly seen depressed mood associated with Alzheimer's disease?

Although in a limited number of cases Prozac does not seem to affect the depressed mood of Alzheimer's patients, the older antidepressants have been used extensively with some positive results.

Is it safe to take Prozac while being treated for medical conditions other than those specifically discussed in this chapter?

A general principle of medicine is that when treating any patient for a depressive disorder, where there is also a coexisting major medical problem, extra caution and lower dosages should be used with the antidepressant medication. Similarly, patients with a history of allergic sensitivities to other medications should be watched carefully while being given Prozac. If a rash occurs, Prozac should be decreased or discontinued.

Can diabetics safely use Prozac if depressed?

The use of Prozac in diabetic patients may alter the blood sugar control. Hypoglycemia, an abnormally low amount of glucose in the blood, has been reported in diabetic patients taking Prozac, and discontinuing therapy has occasionally produced hyperglycemia, an abnormally high concentration of sugar in the blood.

There is insufficient data to prove that Prozac alone can cause all of these changes in blood sugar, and so most diabetic patients may be treated safely with Prozac. However, when initiating therapy with Prozac and later when discontinuing its use, it is important to keep a close watch on blood glucose levels and adjust insulin three to four times a day accordingly. My depressed diabetic patients have done extremely well on long-term Prozac.

Is it safe to take Prozac and other medications at the same time?

The more medications a person is taking, the greater the chance for potential problems. Drugs interact. So whenever a second medication is in the body, it should mean extra caution on the part of the physician and patient. Potential drug interactions should always be researched by the treating physician.

What should patients and physicians do about Prozac in the case of hospitalization for medical treatment or surgery?

Patients who are undergoing medical treatment or surgery while taking Prozac need to be cautious, especially if the medical treatment or surgery involves renal or liver function, because Prozac is excreted by the kidneys and metabolized by the liver.

If at all possible, it is advisable to stop taking Prozac (and any other antidepressant drug) several weeks before a scheduled surgery and to begin slowly reinstating the drug only when the recuperating patient has started to take food and fluids by mouth.

Can Prozac be safely taken during pregnancy? Will it harm my unborn child?

A patient on Prozac who is pregnant or intends to become pregnant should notify her physician immediately. While studies in animals show that even with a dose of Prozac ten times larger than what is normally considered the maximum there is no evidence of harm to the fetus, adequate well-controlled studies have not yet been done with pregnant women. Since animal studies are not always predictive of what occurs in humans, it is a safer policy to avoid Prozac (and other antidepressants) while trying to conceive, or to withdraw from it if already pregnant. Only if a severe depressive relapse occurs should Prozac or other antidepressants be considered during pregnancy.

However, one substance requires a specific warning: lithium. Most studies, except one recent publication, have shown that lithium therapy throughout the first trimester of pregnancy and beyond may be associated with birth defects, especially in the cardiovascular system. Consequently, women who are taking lithium are advised to discontinue immediately if they are actively trying to become pregnant or have just conceived.

Has Prozac had any effect on male or female reproduction or fertility?

Limited studies have shown no effect on reproductive functioning or fertility in both sexes. Men are able to take Prozac throughout their reproductive life without any harmful effects on sperm count.

Is breast-feeding contraindicated while taking Prozac? What about post-partum depression?

Yes. Like many drugs, Prozac and its metabolite, norfluoxetine, are excreted in the mother's milk. Since it is uncertain what temporary or final effect this would have on an infant, mothers who intend to nurse their babies should not take Prozac or other antidepressants. Prozac and other antidepressants are effective in treating post-partum depression, but mothers who take these medications should not nurse.

Does Prozac cause seizures?

During the course of the premarketing development of Prozac, a total of twelve patients out of more than six thousand experienced convulsions or seizures. This is a rate of 0.2%, similar to that associated with other antidepressants that have been used safely over the past thirty years.

Although it has not been established whether Prozac served as a triggering mechanism in those cases, patients with a history of seizures or epilepsy clearly need to be cautious, even if they are already taking antiepileptic medications. Before beginning Prozac or any antidepressant drug, they must have a full neurologic workup including an EEG. Both physician and neurologist must be aware of the patient's intention to take Prozac. If the decision is made to go ahead, several precautions should be taken:

- Prozac must be given in smaller doses than usual at the beginning.

- Blood levels of the anticonvulsants must be monitored both at the beginning and as the dosage is raised.

- Serial EEGs must be taken throughout, and especially at the beginning of treatment.

What medical conditions may result in symptoms that confound psychopharmacologists and make it difficult to diagnose major depression?

Hypothyroidism is the most common medical condition associated with depression. Many central nervous system illnesses and injuries, including syphilis, central nervous system tumors, multiple sclerosis, stroke, and head trauma are also accompanied by secondary depressed mood. Hyperthyroidism, Cushing's disease, hyperparathyroidism, and certain vitamin deficiencies can be associated with hypomania and in some cases depression.

Certain drugs, including steroids, amphetamines, Ritalin, and over-the-counter appetite suppressants may cause outbursts of mania or hypomania or precipitate depression or withdrawal.

Is it safe to drive the car while on Prozac?

Because several classes of psychoactive medications may at one time or another impair judgment, thinking or motor skills, people who are beginning treatment with any antidepressant should be advised to avoid driving a car or operating hazardous machinery until they and their doctors are reasonably certain that their illness is stabilized and their performance is not affected.

The period for not driving or operating machinery is during the severely depressed phase of the illness.

When the patient has been stabilized, the depression has lifted, and the dosage of the drug has been established, the patient can usually drive.

Does Prozac damage the brain?

No brain damage whatsoever has been detected in animal or human studies, even after Prozac has been given in doses many times higher than that which is normally considered safe.

Can Prozac be used for chronic fatigue syndrome?

Chronic fatigue syndrome is an elusive disease, difficult to diagnose (in part because some doctors don't believe it exists) and difficult to treat or certainly to cure. Its primary symptom, overwhelming tiredness, often accompanied by disturbed sleep, can also be an indication of depression. Antidepressants, which boost energy, counteract depression, and may help to straighten out the sleep cycle, are frequently useful, and several studies have found Prozac to be successful in treating CFS.

Is Prozac helpful in premenstrual syndrome?

Reports indicate that Prozac has dramatically alleviated some premenstrual symptoms in a small group of patients. Some of the symptoms of PMS include irritability, weeping, a depressed or changeable mood swinging from high to low within hours or days, and the feeling of wanting to isolate oneself from others and not participate in outside activities. Given Prozac's highly successful results with dysthymia and depression, it does not seem surprising that premenstrual depression has been reported to be helped considerably by Prozac. However, further studies are needed.

What reports indicate that Prozac may be useful in Raynaud's syndrome?

Raynaud's syndrome is a blanching of the fingers and an arterial constriction that has been reported for some decades in the medical literature. It is basically unresponsive to most treatment modalities, but one or two reports in the recent literature have indicated success with Prozac treatment.

• 6 •

Aggression, Suicide, and Scientology: The Assault Against Prozac

What role does the Church of Scientology play in the negative reports about Prozac?

The attack against Prozac was launched in November 1989 by the Church of Scientology, a group characterized by the *Wall Street Journal* as "a quasi-religious/business/paramilitary organization" and defined by Funk and Wagnall's 1984 *New Comprehensive International Dictionary* as "a religious and psychotherapeutic cult purporting to solve personal problems, cure mental and physical disorders, and increase intelligence." Founded by L. Ron Hubbard, a science fiction writer who died in 1986, Scientology considers its doctrines to be, as the subtitle of Hubbard's book *Dianetics* explains, "the modern science of mental health." After that book's publication in 1950, mental health professionals spoke out against Scientology. Perhaps in retaliation, Scientologists have long counted psychiatrists, psychiatric medications, and pharmaceutical companies among their many enemies. Prozac, a spokesman alleged, was a "killer drug."

Leading the Scientology attack against Prozac is the Citizens Commission on Human Rights (CCHR), a group which was founded by Scientology in 1969 and which had in the past attacked the amphetamine-like drug Ritalin (widely used for helping hyperactive children achieve a normal attention span.) Once the CCHR set its sights on Prozac, it lobbied against it, sent out mass mailings, and, in October 1990, filed a citizen's petition with the Food and Drug Administration requesting the withdrawal of Prozac from the market—only a few months after the FDA reaffirmed Prozac's safety and efficacy as an antidepressant.

As ammunition, the CCHR made extensive use of an article published in February 1990 in the *American Journal of Psychiatry* by several Boston psychiatrists. The report stated that after two to seven weeks on Prozac, six out of 172 high-risk mental patients who had not been responsive to other drugs became preoccupied with violent, obsessive suicidal thoughts, and that two of them tried (without success) to kill themselves.

Nothing about this was in the least extraordinary to psychiatrists who are familiar with and treat depression. Depressed people are often suicidal: it's a symptom of the disease. About 15% of patients with diagnosed depression eventually commit suicide; about 80% of all patients who commit suicide or make a serious attempt to do so are depressed. At the time and now, most leading psychopharmacologists in the United States felt that it was not a surprise that a few of the deeply depressed patients in the Boston study were suicidal. In addition, four of the six were taking other medications (in one case, *five* other medications). It was also noted that, although none of these patients seemed suicidal when they began taking Prozac, five of the six had had suicidal thoughts in the past.

Nonetheless, because serotonin, the neurotransmitter Prozac specifically affects, may be linked with aggression, there was reason for concern. It was speculated that, in a few instances, Prozac might "tip the balance in the wrong direction, toward violence and aggression."

When the article came to the attention of the CCHR, they took the figures, which were based on a small group of nonresponsive mental patients, and extrapolated them to the entire population. Using the article's statistics, they asserted not only that "up to 140,000 people in the United States have become violent and suicidal by Prozac" but also that Prozac could easily promote killing sprees, a prediction they backed up with one unique story of mass murderer Joseph Wesbecker. In 1989, Wesbecker attacked his co-workers at the Standard Gravure printing plant in Louisville, Kentucky. Using an AK-47 assault rifle, he killed eight, wounded twelve, and then shot himself.

Why did he do this? Speaking on the "Phil Donahue Show," Dennis Clarke, president of the CCHR, announced that he did it because he was taking Prozac. Before that, Clarke said, Wesbecker "had no history of violence."

However, as the *Wall Street Journal* revealed in April 1991, this was completely untrue. Wesbecker had made twelve previous suicide attempts, had often talked of killing his employers, and had accumulated a collection of guns, which he regularly practiced shooting—all *before* he started taking Prozac.

The attack on Prozac was well under way when, on May 6, 1991, *Time* magazine ran a cover story entitled "Scientology: The Cult of Greed." The

Church of Scientology struck back with a $3 million ad campaign in *USA Today* that suggested that *Time* had attempted to forward Hitler and included an attack against Eli Lilly, the manufacturer of Prozac.

The result of all this? Sales of Prozac, by then a full 25 percent of the antidepressant market, slipped to 21 percent. In a dozen cases around the nation, defense attorneys argued that their clients were not responsible for their actions because they had been taking Prozac. Even more disturbing to me and other psychiatrists, many patients decided on their own to discontinue the drug, with the predictable result that their depression worsened and in some cases their suicidal thoughts became more intense. Worst of all, some patients needed to be hospitalized as a result of going off their medication.

In July 1991, the FDA rejected the CCHR petitions, once again reaffirming the safety of Prozac. Two months later, the FDA Advisory Committee and an independent scientific advisory committee unanimously announced that Prozac and other antidepressants do not cause suicide or violent behavior; in fact, Prozac seemed to protect against violent behavior, and large clinical trials indicate that patients taking Prozac are actually less suicidal than those taking a placebo or other antidepressant drugs.

Nonetheless, the CCHR and a handful of attorneys have continued this campaign against Prozac, twisting the scientific data, misrepresenting the clinical experience, and discouraging patients from taking a drug that has been accepted in more than sixty-three countries around the world as a safe and effective way to treat depression. The anti-Prozac campaign has been thoroughly discredited by the FDA, the American Psychiatric Association, and all leading medical authorities. Unfortunately, the ultimate victims of the disinformation campaign are the patients, their families, and the medical profession.

As of 1994, have there been any court decisions granting any negative claims of Prozac's effects on patients?

As of January 1994, 78 suits against Eli Lilly have been dismissed and 160 others have been filed with accusations ranging from charges that Prozac causes rashes to allegations that the drug led to violent, bizarre death.

So far, not a single court has said that Prozac caused suicide or violent behavior in any of the cases brought to trial. Indeed, although approximately a hundred cases are still pending, fifty-one cases have already been dismissed.

One such case is that of Bonnie Leitsch, a Louisville woman who was the national director of the Prozac Survivors Support Group, another organization opposed to Prozac. In November 1990, she brought a $150 million lawsuit against Eli Lilly and Company, claiming that after she started taking Prozac as a "pick-me-up" prescribed by her doctor, she became hostile, argumentative, and impulsive, developed violent thoughts, and for the first time in her life tried to commit suicide. "I wanted to die," she said. "That seemed to be the only answer. Death was the only escape from Prozac." She repeated this dramatic story not only in court but also on "Geraldo" and "Phil Donahue" and "60 Minutes." The case was dismissed when it turned out that Leitsch had taken an overdose of sleeping pills in 1960, had a history of depression in her medical records dating from 1976, when her stepdaughter was shot to death in a gas station robbery, and had recently endured the suicide of her 21-year-old daughter.

So what caused her to try to take her own life? Eli Lilly representatives maintained that it was her disease: depression.

The FDA continues to proclaim Prozac's safety as an antidepressant and has consistently refused to list any warning in the insert package regarding possible suicidal or violent impulses resulting from taking the drug.

Are there any negative reports about Prozac in the scientific literature?

Sure there are. Like any other drug, Prozac doesn't always alleviate depression. Sometimes it doesn't work. And as with other antidepressants, tranquilizers, and antipsychotic drugs, a few isolated reports in the scientific literature indicate that Prozac sometimes produces unusual adverse side effects or induces manic symptoms or other medical or psychiatric conditions. This is the nature of medication; it is no more true of Prozac than of any of the other antidepressants that have been safely used over the past three to four decades.

Is there any link at all between Prozac and suicide?

Patients who take antidepressants are often suicidal to begin with, and they continue to be at risk as the antidepressant agent is escalated. Eighty-six published and unpublished reports claim that in a small minority of patients, Prozac, like other antidepressants, is associated with an increased propensity toward suicidal thoughts.

The reasons for this are unclear, but one commonly held hypothesis is that during the first few weeks of treatment, the antidepressant is thought to boost the patient's energy before it alters his or her mood, with the result that a patient who may have previously been too slowed down by depression to do anything dangerous can now act on impulse rather than remain in a state of lethargy and immobilization.

A number of studies indicate that in the retarded depressed patient—that is, the patient whose thoughts and movements are slowed down or retarded by the depression—the potential for suicide may temporarily increase as the depression lifts. Reports of this phenomenon have circulated in the psychiatric literature for decades.

Another possible explanation is that in a small number of depressed suicidal patients, the administration of Prozac increases anxiety, which could conceivably push the patient over the edge. This increased anxiety and recklessness can be easily monitored by a trained psychopharmacologist, and if necessary, the patient can be hospitalized. Most depression experts agree that when a depressed patient complains of active suicidal thoughts, it is a psychiatric emergency and hospitalization is immediately needed. This is not something to fear. As William Styron wrote in his 1990 memoir of depression, *Darkness Visible,* "The hospital was my salvation."

How common are suicidal acts?

In 1991, a total of 30,810 people killed themselves, making suicide the eighth leading cause of death in the United States. Provisional data indicate that fewer people killed themselves in 1992, dropping suicide a notch on the ladder of death. As of this writing, suicide appears to be the ninth leading cause of death, right behind a new entry in the top eight: HIV infection.

But regardless of the precise figures, the likelihood is strong that far more people than reported actually died by their own hands. Because there is still a stigma against suicide, not all self-inflicted deaths are so labeled, and many forms of suicide, such as single-car accidents and death through drug abuse, are neither acknowledged nor identified as such.

Moreover, the number of people who attempt suicide without success is thought to be fully eight to ten times larger than the number of those who succeed.

How common are suicidal thoughts or feelings among people who are depressed?

Because 15% of patients with bipolar manic depression ultimately commit suicide and the rates for unipolar depression seem to be similar, it would appear that suicidal thoughts are very common.

Between 40% and 60% of patients undergoing an acute episode of major depressive disorder have suicidal thoughts, and an even higher percentage may have a history of suicidal thoughts or wishes. I and many other psychiatrists and psychopharmacologists would go even further, believing that as many as 90% of patients who appear in the psychiatrist's office for the treatment of acute or chronic depression have at some time at least expressed the thought that "I sometimes wish I were dead," or "My family would be better off without me," or "I wish I could go to bed and never wake up," or "I just wish I'd get hit by a car."

What are the major scientific findings regarding any possible connection between Prozac and suicide?

An important study undertaken in 1991 by two Harvard psychiatrists analyzed the data of twenty-seven psychiatrists who had treated a total of 1017 depressed patients with various antidepressants. They recorded how many patients were given each kind of antidepressant; how many patients in each group were suicidal before beginning therapy (the total for the entire population was about 17%); how many in each group were not suicidal; and how many in each group were not suicidal before therapy but became so afterwards. This latter finding was the real purpose of this survey.

The survey reported that:

- of the 231 non-suicidal patients who took Prozac, 3.5% became suicidal after initiating therapy;

- of the 62 non-suicidal patients who took Prozac in combination with a tricyclic antidepressant (TCA), 6.5% became suicidal;

- of the 385 non-suicidal patients who took a TCA alone or in combination with lithium, 1.3% became suicidal;

- of the 63 non-suicidal patients who took a Monoamine Oxidase Inhibitor (MAOI) antidepressant, not one became suicidal;

- of the 101 non-suicidal patients who took other antidepressants, 3% became suicidal.

The differences between these groups were not statistically significant except for the group given a combination of Prozac and a TCA.

An even more extensive study investigating the possible association between Prozac and suicidal acts and thoughts was published in the *British Medical Journal*. This report presented a retrospective analysis of data from seventeen double-blind trials involving 3065 patients with major depressive disorder. (This included data from my original research study on 120 depressed patients.) For five or six weeks, 1765 patients were put on Prozac, 731 received a tricyclic antidepressant, and 569 were given a placebo. These trials clearly showed that Prozac was not associated with an increased risk of suicide or suicidal thoughts. The findings include the following:

- substantial suicidal thinking emerged in 1.2% of the patients taking Prozac, 3.6% of those on a TCA, and 2.6% of those taking a placebo;
- suicidal thinking became worse with 15.3% of those on Prozac, 16.3% of those on a TCA, and 17.9% of those who were given a placebo;
- in most patients, suicidal thinking lessened considerably with both antidepressants. 72.0% improved on Prozac compared to 54.8% on the placebo, and 72.5% improved on the TCA vs. 69.8% on the placebo;
- the pooled incidence of suicidal acts was 0.3% for Prozac, 0.4% for the TCAs, and 0.2% for the placebo;
- none of these differences were considered statistically significant.

Will Prozac make me irritable or angry?

Not according to the evidence collected so far. A limited number of scientific studies has shown that Prozac decreases aggression as well as attacks of anger and rage in depressed patients. However, if hypomanics have mistakenly been given Prozac, they may react by becoming even more irritable and angry, or by developing manic rage and psychosis.

One interesting study looked at the prevalence of sudden, intense bursts of anger among 127 outpatients with major depression at the Massachusetts General Hospital. After being given a variety of questionnaires testing for anger, hostility, and depression, 44% of these patients were identified as having anger attacks. These anger attacks were accompanied by a constellation of symptoms, among which were feeling out of control; feeling like attacking others; rapid heart rate; hot flashes; fear, panic, or anxiety; and shaking or trembling. The patients who reported these anger attacks were also significantly more anxious and hostile.

After eight weeks of treatment with 20 mg of Prozac a day, the anger attacks disappeared in 71% of the patients who had reported them in the beginning of the study.

The researchers also found that 6% of those who did not report anger attacks initially did report them after eight weeks of treatment.

Has Prozac been associated with violent behavior?

We live in a violent society. Over 4 million individuals in the United States are victims of violence each year. Data from the National Center for Health Statistics report 8.7 premature deaths due to homicide per 100,000 people in the United States in 1985, making homicide the second leading cause of injury or death among children. Furthermore, homicide is the leading cause of death among black males ages 15 through 24, and the third leading cause, after motor vehicle injury and suicide, among white males 15 to 24 years of age. Nonfatal violence is even more widespread. In 1985, some 113 violent interactions occurred for every 1000 married couples, and 620 violent interactions occurred for every 1000 children and their parents.

Despite the fact that violence is so common in the population as a whole, violent events have rarely been reported in association with Prozac. Once in a while, a patient on Prozac has been hauled into court for some harmful act. Nonetheless, in every one of those instances, Prozac has been exonerated of responsibility. Not a single one of the criminals who have come to court armed with the so-called Prozac defense has succeeded in convincing a judge or jury that the crime was committed because the defendant was on Prozac. In all of the cases, the criminal has been convicted and the medication acquitted: a 100% victory for the pharmaceutical company.

Can Prozac make me more anxious or high-strung?

Some patients complain that they feel "revved up," anxious, agitated, or "jittery" on Prozac, in which case the dose should be lowered.

What are the effects of Prozac on patients who mutilate themselves?

It is disturbing that about 4% of patients in mental hospitals have used razor blades, knives, or broken glass to slash themselves on the arms or legs or body. (That number is approximately fifty times larger than in the population as a whole.) Of these people, most are in their twenties, three out of four are women, and over half have tried to commit suicide. They generally cut themselves repeatedly, over a period of years. This is another area where Prozac and other SSRI antidepressants offer promise to real help. A number of cases have been reported where patients suffering from compulsive self-mutilation and obsessive-compulsive disorder responded well to Prozac and other new antidepressant medications.

How do you make a patient feel comfortable about taking Prozac despite the negative publicity that it has received?

I begin by pointing out to my patients that the Food and Drug Administration has rejected attempts to remove Prozac from the market, rejected the accusations that associated Prozac with suicidal or homicidal thoughts, rejected a petition requesting that the Prozac label be changed to include a warning about suicidal or violent behavior, and repeatedly affirmed Prozac's safety and efficacy as an antidepressant.

I add that the FDA's decision to support Prozac was supported by the National Mental Health Association and by the American Psychiatric Association.

I recommend that my patients read this book. I also make sure that my patients know that I will monitor their progress meticulously. I require my patients to come into the office once a week for the first month, then bi-weekly, and eventually monthly.

Finally, I briefly summarize my clinical experience with Prozac to my patients. I have used Prozac for over nine years, from the time when it was an investigational new compound undergoing medical trials to the present. I have given Prozac to a large number of depressed patients alone or in combination with lithium or other drugs. I have concluded that it is a highly effective, very safe antidepressant.

I have never had a depressed patient who became violent on Prozac, although some depressed patients are angry at the beginning of treatment. Untreated hypomanic and manic patients can be violent.

I have never had a depressed patient commit suicide on Prozac, although many of my depressed patients have suicidal thoughts at the beginning of treatment or have had them in the past, and a number of them have tried suicide.

Since I first started using Prozac with depressed patients, I have, however, seen hundreds of people with a variety of conditions who, with the help of this drug, have turned their lives around, moving out of their depression into wellness. Essentially, they feel fine.

• 7 •

Prozac and Other Medications: The Psychiatrist's Pharmacopeia

Do antidepressants and lithium really make a difference in the treatment of depression?

They make a tremendous difference. Correctly prescribed and taken, antidepressants generate major improvement in 65% to 80% of depressed patients. Along with lithium and antianxiety medications, the new antidepressants have successfully treated millions of patients worldwide and enabled them to function normally or at least better. No longer need lives be wasted in devastating depression or in destructive uncontrolled manic episodes.

Moreover, these medications have an effect that extends beyond the lives of those for whom they are prescribed. Depression is not only a personal and family/societal problem, it is also a problem that results in lost time on the job, divorce, hospitalization, suicide, secondary alcoholism, and drug addiction. Depression and other mood disorders waste lives— and money. According to a recent study, the annual costs of depression in the United States total approximately $43.7 billion.

As William Styron remarks in *Darkness Visible,* depression is a "true wimp of a word for such a major illness." Depressed people visit their doctors three times as often as do patients without a psychiatric disorder and they spend more days in bed than do people with hypertension, diabetes, arthritis, and back pain.

Yet, with a frequency that is shocking—50% to 60% of the time in primary care settings, 60% of the time in HMOs—the disorder goes undiagnosed. This is tragic, because when depression is recognized and appropriately treated with medication and/or therapy, it can be eliminated most of the time—or at least controlled.

If Prozac is as good as everyone says it is, why do doctors still prescribe other drugs for depression?

Many physicians and psychopharmacologists feel comfortable with tricyclic antidepressants (TCAs) and monoamine oxidase inhibitors (MAOIs) because for over thirty-five years they have prescribed them with great success for millions of patients. It is true that these drugs have more side effects than Prozac and the other new SSRIs, but patients can often tolerate the side effects without undue complaints if educated in what to expect: dry mouth, constipation, sometimes a little dizziness, mild sexual difficulties. These side effects are annoying but not terrible, and by and large, these older antidepressants have worked well. Thus, many physicians are reluctant to prescribe a new drug, despite the miraculous claims that may accompany it. Faced with a depressed patient, cautious, conservative physicians and psychopharmacologists often turn to the old medications first. If the patient cannot tolerate the side effects or if the dosage, when escalated to the top, does not bring the patient out of the depression, then they may try one of the new SSRI antidepressants, Wellbutrin, or Effexor.

Finally, many psychiatrists prefer to prescribe the older drugs whose long-term effects are predictable rather than a new drug whose long-term safety is still unknown.

Despite the hesitation of so many conservative physicians, the number of psychiatrists using the old battery of ten to fifteen antidepressants has eroded every year since Prozac was launched.

What has been the major impact of Prozac on the treatment of depression, manic depression, dysthymia, and personality disorders?

Because the clinical efficacy of Prozac in depression is at least equal to the standard antidepressants, and because the side effects of Prozac are so much milder, the major impact of Prozac has been that patients, families, and physicians have preferred it and the newer drugs to most of the previously used drugs. Its safety and efficacy, in combination with the flood of publicity, both good and bad, it has received since it was first introduced to the American market in 1987, have made Prozac the number one best-selling antidepressant in the United States. In 1993, its sales reached $1.2 billion, exceeding the sales of all previously used antidepressant drugs both nationally and internationally.

What are the main advantages of Prozac over the previously prescribed antidepressants?

The main advantages of Prozac, compared to both the tricyclics and the MAOIs, are that it has minimal side effects, is not lethal in overdose, and has much milder effects on the cardiovascular system. Specifically, it does not lower blood pressure, and it causes a far lower incidence of dry mouth, dizziness, constipation, or blurred vision than do most of the TCAs and MAOIs.

Is Prozac only a fad, like Miltown, Librium, Valium and Xanax have been in the sixties, seventies, and eighties? In what ways is it different?

No, I don't believe so, although some critics have claimed that Prozac is simply another happy pill, replacing the popular drugs of recent decades. There is a difference, however. Miltown, Librium, Valium, and Xanax are all classed as minor tranquilizing drugs with habituating properties. They have been and are being prescribed for anxiety disorders and, in some cases, panic attacks.

Prozac belongs to an entirely different group of drugs classified as antidepressants, with an entirely different mechanism of action and without the habit-forming properties that proved so troublesome with the antianxiety drugs listed above.

But even aside from these differences, there has never before been a fad for an antidepressant drug like the one that has accompanied Prozac. Other drug fads have promised that you'll feel better and more relaxed. Prozac's reputation promises not just that you'll feel better but that you'll feel, seem, and be different. It has been touted not only as a useful treatment for depression but as an aid for non-depressed people who want a "personality change" or just want to be happier.

The major reason for this reputation is that the media have blown up the usefulness of Prozac and have implied promises for it that extend far beyond the diagnostic conditions of major depressive disorder and obsessive-compulsive disorder, for which it is FDA approved. Clinical trials to date simply do not warrant the exaggerated claims for this new compound as a panacea for all psychiatric and personality problems of the "worried well."

Just because the claims are exaggerated doesn't mean that they are completely false. Although many patients feel improved with Prozac, approximately 10% feel rapidly and distinctly better than their usual selves. This latter group—and it's possible to predict who they will be with a reasonable degree of certainty—sometimes claim to feel better than they've ever felt before. Prozac is not a cure-all, but it is likely that the claims that Prozac can make a person more outgoing, less fearful, and more self-confident are indeed true. These claims are in fact true for all antidepressant drugs. Fear, uncertainty and a lack of self-confidence are standard symptoms of depression. When the depression lifts for any reason, these symptoms disappear. I have seen this happen with many of my depressed and introverted, shy patients.

Does Prozac differ from other antidepressant drugs in the way it influences personality?

When a person's mood shifts, the outward picture of his or her personality and behavior also changes as a consequence. Although no scientific evidence indicates that Prozac is different from other antidepressant drugs in its effect on primary personality traits, many psychiatrists, patients, and families have made claims of Prozac's remarkable ability to change a patient's outlook, energy level, and mood in such a way that the entire personality *seems* changed. It often produces a general brightening, optimism, and assertiveness that had not been present for months or years before. Other antidepressant drugs, while capable of producing similar effects and rates of success, simply have not generated the same amount of press coverage. Despite the very similar rates of success that some other antidepressant drugs have had, the media and the medical profession have not emphasized them so prominently.

What are the differences between drugs of abuse and nonhabit-forming drugs like Prozac, which often must be taken for many years, even though the acute depression has been removed by the drug?

Drugs of abuse, including amphetamines, sleeping pills, and most minor tranquilizers have two properties in common: tolerance, or the need to take increasingly larger doses of the drug to achieve the same effect; and withdrawal, a rebound of mild to severe symptoms and side effects that occurs upon stopping the drug. All antidepressant drugs including Prozac are non-habit forming and do not have either of these characteristics.

Can I take normal over-the-counter drugs like aspirin, Advil, Tylenol, and Anacin while I'm taking Prozac?

Yes. There are no negative interactions to be expected with these drugs.

What about other over-the-counter or prescription drugs?

Patients on Prozac should inform the physician if they plan to take any prescription or over-the-counter nonprescription drugs. However, in clinical trials, the following drugs all appear to be safe:

- analgesics
- antacids
- antibiotics
- antihistamines

- beta-adrenergic blockers for cardiac disease
- cathartics
- chloral hydrate
- H_2-blockers such as Zantac and Tagamet
- oral contraceptives
- thyroid hormones.

What about marijuana, cocaine, LSD, or other similar drugs?

These illegally obtained mood-altering drugs are all completely contraindicated for patients taking Prozac—and this would be true even if they were legal. Taken with or without Prozac, these drugs can cause uncontrolled highs, severe depression, and psychotic states in some people. For patients already prone to these reactions, the risk is high if an antidepressant drug like Prozac is added.

What medications, besides psychiatric drugs, must be used cautiously or not at all while taking Prozac?

Theoretically, two drugs may require particular caution until all of the data are in: the blood thinner Coumadin (warfarin) and some Digitalis-related drugs taken for heart failure. Those drugs, like Prozac and other SSRIs, are tightly bound to plasma proteins. Administering Prozac along with either of these medications may *in theory* alter their plasma concentrations, with potentially serious results.

However, contrary to these expectations, a single clinical scientific study looking at the interactions between Prozac, Coumadin, Diuril, Orinase, Valium, and diazepam found that Prozac had little effect on the actions of those drugs. Further drug interaction studies are needed.

What drugs prescribed for medical purposes sometimes precipitate major depression or dysthymia?

Drugs that sometimes lead to major depression and dysthymia include:

- antihypertensive drugs such as reserpine, methyldopa, propranolol, guanethidine, hydralazine, and clonidine
- anti-infective drugs such as Cycloserine
- anti-Parkinson drugs including Levodopa, amantadine, and carbidopa
- corticosteroids
- estrogen and progesterone
- the anticancer drugs Vincristine and Vinblastine.

Similarly, some reports have attempted to associate the onset of depression with the taking of minor or major tranquilizers.

What antidepressants are available for depressed patients in the United States and abroad?

The most important antidepressants can be divided into several main categories:

- tricyclic antidepressants (TCAs)
- monoamine oxidase inhibitors (MAOIs)
- selective serotonin reuptake inhibitors (SSRIs)
- lithium
- structurally unrelated compounds.

How do these medications differ?

Tricyclic antidepressants (TCAs), so-called because they have three rings in their chemical structure, work in the brain by making certain that the neurotransmitter norepinephrine (NE) and, to a lesser extent, serotonin (SE), remain in the synapse between nerve fibers rather than being taken back up into the nerve cell itself. The end result of this is that the amount of neurotransmitter in the synapse increases, thereby allowing the flow of nerve impulses to return to normal. This is associated with an antidepressant response in the patient.

First-generation tricyclics include:

- the first TCA, imipramine (Tofranil), which was introduced in 1958
- amitriptyline (Elavil)
- desipramine (Norpramin)
- nortriptyline (Pamelor)
- protriptyline (Vivactil)
- clomipramine (Anafranil)
- trimipramine (Surmontil)
- the European medication amineptine (Survector).

Although side effects vary from drug to drug and person to person, the side effects generally associated with TCAs include dry mouth, constipation, blurred vision, weight gain, an increased heart rate, drowsiness, urinary retention, memory problems, impotence, decreased blood pressure and dizziness when standing up. It generally takes between 7 and 15 days before the drug begins to have an antidepressant effect.

Related medications called tetracyclics include maprotiline (Ludiomil), amoxapine (Asendin), and the European drug mianserin (Bolvidon).

Monoamine oxidase inhibitors (MAOIs) work by

preventing the breakdown of the neurotransmitter hormones norepinephrine and serotonin, which in turn has the effect of increasing the amount of those substances in the synapses.

MAOIs include:

- incarboxazid (Marplan)
- phenelzine (Nardil)
- tranylcypromine (Parnate).

Besides such side effects as restlessness, dizziness, and weight gain, MAOIs have one unique problem. You have to be very careful what you eat while taking an MAOI. Ordinary foods that contain *tyramine* including—but not limited to—cheese, Chianti wine, yogurt, lima beans, pickled herring, smoked meats, liver, and large amounts of caffeine or chocolate can trigger a sudden rise in blood pressure that has been known to cause blood vessels in the brain to burst, the so-called cheese effect. A stroke or even death can be the outcome. A related MAOI is the European drug Deprenyl, which is marketed in the United States as an anti-Parkinson drug, not an antidepressant. It requires less attention to dietary restriction.

Selective serotonin reuptake inhibitors (SSRIs) block the uptake only of serotonin, thereby causing it to increase in the nerve synapse. SSRIs include:

- fluoxetine (Prozac)
- sertraline (Zoloft)
- paroxetine (Paxil)
- fluvoxamine (Luvox)

- nefazadone (Serzone)
- citalopram (under development).

These drugs relieve depression as effectively the TCAs and MAOIs, but their side effect profile is considerably milder.

Lithium, although primarily used as a mood stabilizer with manic-depressive disorders, can also play an important prophylactic role in recurrent unipolar depression and even a therapeutic role in major depression when it is added to an antidepressant as a step-up treatment. It comes in these generic forms under various trade names:

- lithium carbonate
- slow-release lithium carbonate
- lithium citrate syrup (liquid).

Structurally unrelated compounds used for the treatment of depression include a number of other medications, such as:

- trazodone (Deseryl)
- buproprion (Wellbutrin)
- venlafaxine (Effexor).

Can Prozac be used simultaneously with the tricyclic antidepressants (TCAs)?

Although this has not been studied sufficiently, Prozac is frequently given in clincial practice with small doses of TCAs. Adding Prozac to a TCA has occasionally led to an increase—even a doubling—of the previously stable blood level of the TCA. This requires more study.

Is it safe to take Prozac with monoamine oxidase inhibitors (MAOIs)?

No. Monoamine oxidase inhibitors (MAOIs) and Prozac just don't mix. A few patients who have taken both drugs simultaneously have had severe reactions that include confusion, sweating, shivering, muscle spasms, tremors, and restlessness, as well as symptoms of rigidity, hyperthermia, rapid fluctuations of pulse and blood pressure, extreme agitation, delirium, coma, and in eight cases, death. Even patients who stopped taking Prozac and then immediately started up on an MAOI have had these reactions.

A patient who wants to switch to Prozac from an MAOI must allow fourteen days to elapse after discontinuing MAOI treatment before the MAOI is completely out of the system. Only then can Prozac be safely tried.

A patient who wants to go in the other direction, ceasing treatment with Prozac and beginning treatment with an MAOI, must wait even longer. Because Prozac and its major breakdown product, norfluoxetine, remain in the body for a long time, *a minimum* of five weeks is needed after discontinuing Prozac before MAOI treatment can commence.

Can Prozac be used with second generation antidepressants such as Desyrel (trazodone), Ludiomil (maprotiline), and Asendin (amoxapine)?

Caution should be used if any of these drugs is taken with Prozac, and small doses should be given until further scientific evidence is forthcoming as to the combined safety. Enough research just hasn't been done, but to date I have used the combination and it appears safe.

Is Prozac a substitute for lithium?

In no way is Prozac a substitute for lithium. Prozac is an antidepressant, and lithium is a mood stabilizer. Prozac has potent properties of relieving mild to major depression and perhaps prevents recurrent depression as well. At the same time, Prozac may induce mania or hypomania in patients who have a bipolar manic depressive history but are not taking lithium.

Lithium, on the other hand, has a mild antidepressant effect in depressive disorders, a strong antimanic effect, and, finally, a prophylactic effect on both the highs and lows of bipolar illness and the lows of recurrent depression.

Although lithium is most successful in controlling manic highs, it does not always eradicate the depressive phases of bipolar disorders. In those instances, lithium and Prozac or any of the other antidepressants can be used in combination for long-term maintenance. I have used this combination in many patients over the last six to seven years.

Has Prozac proven to be as effective long-term as lithium?

Not yet. Lithium, which offered the first effective, long-term treatment for manic depression, has been readily available in the United States since 1973 and was used as early as 1948 in Australia, 1954 in Denmark, and a few years later in England and Canada. Prozac was introduced to the American market in 1987. Consequently, lithium has been clinically evaluated for a much longer time in many more centers and studies around the world. Its uses are known. In many ways, Prozac is still being explored. I believe that when its successes and failures are more fully defined, it will prove, like lithium, to be a breakthrough drug for specific, identifiable populations of psychiatric patients.

Under what circumstances can Prozac be used with lithium?

Increasingly, lithium and Prozac are being used together, usually in cases of bipolar manic depression where lithium alone has not controlled the depressive side of the illness and in cases of recurrent unipolar depression for long-term stabilization. (Other antidepressants have also been used with or without lithium to control recurrent depression.) Lithium can also be used as a step-up treatment when TCA, MAOI, or SSRI antidepressants don't seem to be working on their own.

Tens of thousands of bipolar patients in the United States and abroad are safely using Prozac with lithium. Frequent monitoring is necessary because there have been infrequent reports of increased or decreased lithium levels, which may or may not be related to the Prozac.

Finally, patients diagnosed with recurrent schizoaffective disorder with prominent depressive component have sometimes been treated for long-term stabilization with a combination of lithium, Prozac, and an anti-psychotic medication. Thyroid medication may also be included in the regimen as a step-up treatment for the depression component of the illness.

Are there any long-term complications associated with Prozac or with the combination of Prozac and lithium?

No long-term complications of Prozac are known to date, although the full story is not in, since Prozac has only been on the market approximately seven years. Only after twenty or thirty years of closely observing a large number of patients taking an antidepressant can one make conclusions about any of its potential long-term complications.

Long-term effects of lithium have been identified, however. They include the possibility of goiter or altered thyroid function in a small percentage of patients. Some long-term lithium patients with previous kidney impairment tend to lose an even greater degree of kidney function over time. These patients should either switch to a lithium alternative such as Tegretol or Depakote, or be maintained on smaller doses of long-term lithium. I monitor kidney function every one or two months in these cases and I also consult a nephrologist.

Can Prozac be used safely in combination with Tegretol (carbamazepine) or Depakote (valproic acid), and under what conditions is it called for?

Bipolar and schizoaffective patients often have psychotic features that lithium alone has failed to control. In these cases, Tegretol or Depakote may be substituted for lithium or added to it. An antipsychotic may also be needed. If the depression is still moderate to severe, an antidepressant such as Prozac must be added to stabilize the illness. Patients receiving Tegretol or Depakote may have Prozac added in combination with the usual concerns for idiosyncratic reactions.

Can Prozac be used in combination with major tranquilizers such as Thorazine, Mellaril, Trilafon, Stelazine, Haldol, Loxapine, Navane, and Prolixin?

To date, there are no contraindications for using these major tranquilizers in combination with Prozac. However, doses of these drugs, when used in combination, should be started low and escalated slowly and cautiously. Usually an anti-Parkinson

drug such as cogentin, artane, benadryl, or kemadrine should be added to counteract the side effects
of these major tranquilizers.

**Can Prozac be used in conjunction with habit-
forming minor tranquilizers such as Valium
(diazepam), Xanax (alprazolam), Ativan (lorazepam)
or Klonopin (clonazepam)? What about tranquilizers that are not habit-forming, such as Buspar
(buspirone)?**

There are no known contraindications to using
Prozac with these minor tranquilizers, both habit-
forming and nonhabit-forming. However, all the
data is not in. Habit-forming medications should be
used sparingly. Caution is warranted in combining
buspirone, a non-habit forming antianxiety drug,
with Prozac due to a few reports of hypomanic reactions.

**Can Prozac be used safely with hypnotics (sleeping
pills) including Restoril, Dalmane, Halcion, chloral
hydrate, and barbiturates?**

There are no known contraindications for using
Prozac in combination with any of these sleeping
pills. Remember, however, that all of them have
habit-forming properties and cross-addictive tolerance with alcohol. Alcoholics should not be given
these hypnotics, and nonalcoholics should be given
low doses for short periods of time to avoid doctor-
induced addicions to these substances.

How compliant are most patients taking Prozac?

It is a mysterious fact of human nature that patients are generally *not* compliant. They don't take
their full dose of penicillin, they forget to bring their
blood pressure pills on weekend trips, and they self-
regulate, increasing or decreasing the dosage, often

by at least 40%. Studies have shown that only 50% of the time do patients take their medications as prescribed. And in some surveys the number is as high as 93%.

Patients on Prozac are much more compliant than those on other antidepressants. In the combined data of all the Prozac clinical trials, patients taking tricyclic antidepressants stopped taking their medication at approximately twice the rate as those on Prozac. The main reasons for this difference are that Prozac has fewer side effects than other antidepressants and that patients on Prozac need to swallow only one or two pills a day on the average, while patients taking TCAs need to take between three and six pills daily.

An additional factor in the antidepressant equation is contact with the doctor. Studies have shown that the longer the period between visits to the physician, the poorer the compliance rate: patients who see the doctor on a weekly basis are more compliant than those with monthly appointments, who are more compliant than those who see the doctor every two to three months. I insist that my well bipolar and unipolar patients see me for monthly monitoring of blood levels of medications, clinical state, and side effects.

How do the other SSRIs compare to Prozac in efficacy, safety, and side effects?

Two recently marketed SSRIs include Zoloft (generic name setraline) and Paxil (paroxetine). Both new drugs appear to be equal to Prozac in efficacy and safety. Like Prozac, Zoloft and Paxil have minimal side effects, compared to the older tricyclics and MAOIs.

Both Zoloft and Paxil have shorter half-lives than Prozac, which suggests that on sudden withdrawal, there is a greater likelihood of producing symptoms than with Prozac, which tapers itself off over a longer period of time.

Evidence indicates that all varieties of sexual side effects occur in approximately one third of all patients taking antidepressant medications, old and new.

How does Prozac compare with Anafranil (clomipramine) in treating obsessive-compulsive disorder (OCD)?

An estimated 5 million Americans are afflicted with obsessive-compulsive disorder, a biologically based syndrome whose symptoms are recurrent and intrusive obsessive thoughts and compulsive, time-consuming behaviors that shape and even dominate the person's life—even though the patient knows these thoughts and behaviors are irrational. The standard drug for treatment of OCD has long been the tricyclic antidepressant Anafranil (clomipramine), but in July 1993, the Food and Drug Administration unanimously approved Prozac as a treatment for OCD.

Once more, Prozac's superiority as a treatment for some patients has much to do with its minor side effects. Anafranil, when taken in the high doses required for OCD (200 to 300 mg a day), often produces severe constipation, dry mouth, thirst, urinary problems, and gastrointestinal complaints. These symptoms do not occur with Prozac except in a extremely mild form on occasion.

Luvox (fluvoxamine), a recently released SSRI approved for treatment of OCD, appears to be as effective as Prozac or Anafronil for this condition. Although not FDA approved for depression in the United States, Luvox has been used for depression in Canada and Europe for several years.

Is Prozac the only antidepressant that doesn't cause weight gain?

No. Some of the newer antidepressants also do not cause patients to gain weight. Among them are Wellbutrin (buproprion), Zoloft (sertraline), Desyrel (trazodone), and Effexor (Venlafaxine).

The impact of this failure to cause weight gain cannot be overestimated. After all, most of the tricyclics and MAOIs are associated with weight gain, and at least a third of patients who have taken lithium carbonate or the two proposed mood stabilizers, Depakote and Tegretol, tend to put on weight. It's not just a few pounds either, although it starts that way. The longer they stay on the drug, the more weight they gain. Often it's enough to convince them to stop taking the antidepressant. One study found that, of those patients who stopped taking a tricyclic antidepressant, 48% made the decision because they were disturbed by the weight gain.

With Prozac, although some cases of weight gain have been recorded, in most cases weight remains constant or patients actually lose a few pounds. This can make all the difference in the world in terms of both compliance and self-esteem. Howver, recent reports indicate that although intial weight loss may occur with all of these drugs, some patients appear to gain it back within three to twelve months.

One patient, Z.N., a successful television writer, told me that ten years ago, before her first depression, she weighed 110 pounds. After a round of antidepressants that included Nardil, Elavil, and lithium, her weight ballooned to 145 pounds and she grew from size 6 to size 12 over a three-year period.

Since starting Prozac a couple of years ago, she has lost a total of twenty-five pounds. Initially she dropped fifteen pounds, then she gained back five, and then slowly, with Prozac and the help of Weight Watchers, lost another fifteen pounds. Prozac is not a miraculous anti-obesity pill; she has worked at losing weight, and she is still dieting. But with Prozac, she has been able to accomplish this feat. With most earlier antidepressants, it wouldn't have been possible. The same effect appears to be possible in some depressed patients taking Zoloft, Paxil, Wellbutrin, and Venlafaxine.

How do Prozac and Wellbutrin compare to other antidepressants?

Prozac and Wellbutrin do not have the same mechanism of action. Wellbutrin works mainly by blocking the uptake of the neurotransmitter dopamine in the brain; Prozac and other SSRIs work by blocking the uptake of serotonin.

Would taking Prozac make me more sensitive to the sun?

No. Major tranquilizers such as Thorazine and Mellaril do have this side effect, but patients who take Prozac do not show any increase in photosensitivity to light or sun. Major tranquilizers are mostly used for schizophrenia, schizoaffective disorder, and during the first ten days of manic psychosis until lithium takes over.

Can Prozac be used concomitantly with electroconvulsive treatment (ECT)?

Preferably not. As of 1993, there were no clinical studies establishing any benefit from the combined use of ECT and Prozac. Worse, there have been rare reports of prolonged seizures in patients on Prozac receiving electroconvulsive (once called electroshock) treatment. Since no benefit has been identified in leaving the patient on Prozac while receiving ECT, it is better to discontinue Prozac (or other antidepressants and lithium) three to ten days before ECT is scheduled.

On the other hand, with highly suicidal patients, deferring ECT until the drug completely leaves the system is ill-advised when the condition is considered life-threatening.

With regard to cost, are there any generic drugs comparable to Prozac on the market?

No. There are no generic drugs in the SSRI category as yet. Prozac's patent runs out in 2001, and the other SSRI compounds that have since appeared on the market, Zoloft and Paxil, have patents that run out several years later. Once the patent for the trade name Prozac expires, the generic drug fluoxetine will be sold at a considerably lower price.

In the meantime, Prozac remains an expensive medication.

Are there generic antidepressant drugs which are less expensive?

Yes. A number of earlier antidepressants whose patents have run out are available in generic form both in the tricyclic and MAOI categories and they are considerably cheaper. According to research studies, many of these medications are just as good as Prozac in terms of relief of depression, but all of them have more adverse side effects.

As a scientist, I am more of a theoretician than an experimenter. I have recently taken Wellbutrin with good results. Do you think Prozac might prove superior?

If you're doing well on Wellbutrin, I'd advise you to stay on it. However, if you really want to try Prozac, first discuss it with your psychiatrist and then, if he or she agrees, try it with an interval of a couple of weeks between the two medications.

A past history of seizures or bulimia is associated with higher incidence of Wellbutrin-induced seizures in depressed patients. Hence, if you have had these disorders, you should not be taking Wellbutrin at all.

• 8 •

Prozac and Personality:
The Role of Genetics

The most exaggerated claim that has been made for Prozac, acknowledging that most psychiatric clinicians and researchers agree on its superb antidepressant effects, is that it can also dramatically alter personality in people without an underlying diagnosable clinical or subclinical depression. According to this popular notion, people who are simply unhappy or don't like themselves can, by taking a Prozac pill, become outgoing, assertive, sociable, and confident: new personalities with altered inner selves, creations of the dubious field of "cosmetic psychopharmacology."

In my experience, this simply does not happen. Most people who are helped by Prozac, whether they were only mildly or seriously depressed, just return to their former, non-depressed selves. But some people *do* seem to undergo a rapid and remarkable metamorphosis. This phenomenon is understandable if one is armed with a full knowledge of the patient's family history and genetic background. The signs that enable one to predict who these hyperresponders might be are all degrees of moodswing, ranging from the subtle highs and lows on one end of the bipolar spectrum to full-blown manic depression, along with what geneticists call behavioral (phenotypic) equivalents of manic depression in the family history, which have been shown scientifically to include alcoholism and drug abuse, suicide, gambling, sociopathy, as well as the less commonly recognized behaviors associated with manic excess such as compulsive buying of things not needed, promiscuity (often bizarre), nonstop socializing, excess telephoning without purpose, and finally, workaholism. Depressed patients whose personal or family histories show these tendencies, even in their most subtle, hardly recognizable forms, are in my opinion the candidates who become Prozac hyperresponders.

Among these hyperresponders (no more than 10% of those taking Prozac), there are basically three types that I classify clinically, according to the patient's predepressive behavior, and genetically, according to the family history:

- *Hyperthymic responders* are patients with depression, ranging from minimal to major, who become energetic, outgoing, assertive, efficient, able to organize and prioritize, and more often than not, able to correct the imbalances in their personal and professional lives once the depression has lifted. After taking Prozac, their depression and anxiety disappear. To all outward appearances, their personalities have changed positively. They feel great, and for good reason. They are their old, energetic, sociable—hyperthymic—selves.

- *Hypomanic responders* go one step beyond the hyperthymic. These depressives develop even more energy on Prozac, need very little sleep, and tend to work and socialize compulsively, often very successfully. Family, friends, and peers at the office who notice their rapid accomplishments and non-stop activities may respond at first with admiration but later with a feeling that something is not quite right, and they may describe these hyperresponders as wired or slightly crazy. Extremely demanding, impatient, and unreasonable, these patients are prone to sudden, intense enthusiasm, irritation that may turn into bursts of anger, and lack of judgment in areas as varied as money management (they overextend themselves financially and often commit fraud), sexuality, driving recklessly, and excesses of all kinds. The hypomanic response to Prozac can be both positive and negative. When a patient on Prozac begins to show signs of hypomania, it can become serious and the dose should be immediately lowered or discontinued. The patient may need lithium, but by this time, many have quit treatment only to take a plane to Monte Carlo or Las Vegas.

● *Manic responders* are clearly recognizable and are extremely rare. They possess an unreasonable degree of energy and may go for days on end without sleep, to be followed by collapse into depression and physical exhaustion. They are expansive, grandiose, or paranoid, and filled with unrealistic schemes and theories. They may call the White House, begin suing everyone around them, or try to buy Trump Tower on Fifth Avenue in New York City. Their minds race, and they may become delusional. Their judgment is disastrous and they are unable to function in the workplace or the home. Many of these people are prone to alcoholism as well. Mania requires hospitalization because it evolves quickly into manic psychosis with its complex paranoid systems, hallucinations, and delusions (many of which involve the F.B.I., the C.I.A, and other institutions). This is an infrequent response to Prozac and other antidepressants, new and old, but when it does occur, it requires emergency hospitalization and treatment. This reaction in most cases can be predicted by the skilled psychopharmacologist and avoided by prior treatment with lithium.

The frequency of this last Prozac hyperresponse has not been adequately studied but I would estimate it to be no more than 2% to 3% of all those taking Prozac, depending on the population being studied. In my clinical experience, the more severe the manic episodes or genetic equivalents in the personal or family history, the more likely one is to get an undesirable hypomanic or manic response with antidepressant agents. When a person comes in with such a family history, even if he or she has never shown signs of hypomanic or manic behavior, the prescribing physician must begin gingerly, with a low dose and weekly monitoring. What you're hoping for is a normal response—i.e., a lifting of depression—or even a hyperthymic response, which some psychiatrists may call transformation. In order for this to happen, the genetic potential has to be there.

But occasionally, a chronically depressed person comes in, quickly becomes a Prozac hyperresponder, and yet seems to have no past or family history of manic depression or its equivalents. I believe that in these instances, the manic depressive gene or genes are there but they are not obvious for three possible reasons.

The first reason is that the family history is incomplete.

The second reason is that in some cases the manic depressive tendency expresses itself in positive attributes rather than in illness. When these fortunate patients talk about their families, there are no suicides, alcoholics, or relatives in mental hospitals. Instead, these people, who may also come out of their depression dramatically, may have another signpost: a family history of outstanding achievements. The same genetically endowed energy that, in the worse cases, leads to manic rages, nonstop talking, and alcoholism, may instead express itself positively through *great* accomplishment.

The third reason that the manic depressive gene or genes may not be easily detected in the family history is that they may essentially be weak or of low penetrance. These patients may come into the office with chronic depression only, lacking in both their own past and their family histories the normal ups of hyperthymia, the questionable highs of hypomania, and the psychotic highs of the manic. In these cases, the tendency to display the up side of the manic depressive gene(s) lies dormant (a gene of low penetrance) until an environmental (in this case, psychopharmacological) stimulus comes along and the personality suddenly blooms for the first time. The patient notices a hyperthymic buoyancy—a "new self"—that was literally never there before. It needed a little extra push before it could manifest itself. It needed an antidepressant drug—in this case, Prozac. These patients, who initially may have been diagnosed with major unipolar depression, dysthymia, or personality disorders, are now reclassified as bipolar III, a diagnosis reserved for those depressed patients who show no personal or familial predisposition towards bipolar disorder until an antidepressant drug allows the inherited but hidden tendency to express itself. Hagop S. Akiskal, M.D., Professor of Psychiatry at the University of Tennessee and a consultant at the National Institute of Mental Health, is the leading theoretician and clinical researcher on this area of subsyndromal mood disorders, temperament, and character.

These hyperresponders—whether they have been

lifted into hyperthymia or pushed too far, into hypomania or mania—feel transformed, or, in the latter case, supertransformed into manic psychosis. If the manic depressive gene(s) is not present to some degree as is most often the case, the response to Prozac will instead be more subdued. The patient does not feel transformed but nonetheless, the depression is no longer there. A restoration to wellness has occurred.

Will Prozac bring out my "true self"?

If by your "true self" you mean your normal nondepressed, nonanxious, functioning self, which you feel is your baseline, the answer is yes, if you are currently depressed, since Prozac relieves the symptoms of depression and returns the person to baseline. Both scientific studies and anecdotal reports support the view that Prozac can in this sense return you to your former self.

Can Prozac change my real personality?

Although some patients and physicians have claimed that Prozac has transformed personality very positively, most scientists who have studied personality, clinical psychopharmacology, and genetics do not know that this is true beyond the obvious personality changes seen in all depressed patients whose emotions and behavior are altered by Prozac and other medications.

Scientists do not have sufficient evidence that pharmacological agents such as Prozac cause actual changes either in character, which is acquired through environmental experience, or in the DNA-encoded traits that make up temperament, which is inherited. Character and temperament are the main components of personality.

We only have anecdotal evidence: individual reports of people who have not merely returned to the way they were before they got depressed (the psychiatric term for this is "premorbid personality") but utterly changed, seemingly expressing traits completely unlike those of the person they used to be. But in fact these traits are not completely foreign to them, as detailed questioning by a depression expert will reveal; they have simply been buried, frequently for a long time, under a thick layer of dysthymia, a milder chronic form of depression that may have gone undiagnosed for months, years, or a lifetime. Nonetheless, it shaped the patient's personality and character development, often with a mixture of "soft symptoms," such as sluggishness, timidity, and anxiety—traits that might be aspects of someone's normal personality but that could also be symptoms of subclinical depression. In the latter case, Prozac can lift the patient into a state of normalcy that he or she hasn't felt for years. Both the patient and other people may then perceive the patient's personality to have changed dramatically.

Essentially, I don't believe you can refashion a person's normal personality with Prozac. Depressive symptoms must be present before obvious changes in behavior and emotions can be brought about with an antidepressant. But when there is a past, often forgotten hypomania, the change may be greater and the patient may interpret this as a "transformed self" or a "new personality."

Do some personality types respond to Prozac better than other types?

Yes. Certain types do seem to respond to Prozac more quickly and more positively. The transformations Prozac causes—and make no mistake, I have observed such transformations in depressed patients over the last thirty years—occur in a particular population. They happen with people who may be depressed and lethargic when they come into my office, but in the past have had often undisclosed periods of higher energy—and the accomplishments to prove it. These patients are *not* diagnosable manic-depressive. But they have a tendency in that direction, with perhaps only one or two symptoms of subclinical depression that affect their personalities and typically send them on a fruitless search for a cure through psychotherapy alone rather than medication. Yet some psychologists and psychiatrists, having failed to detect the subclinical depression or soft bipolar symptoms in the past or family history, misdiagnose these patients as having character or personality disorders only. Psychotherapy consists of focusing on drives and defenses—ignoring the formes frustes symptoms of mood disorders. In short, the correctable symptoms do not get treated.

These people often have a buried past of hyperthymia, a mildly "up" state with brisk energy, buoyant optimism, and an irritable temper. Hyperthymic people get a lot done and normally need only four to six hours' sleep—like President Bill Clinton, who, I would guess, is most likely hyperthymic and constantly on the run. This is not an illness; it is an asset. These people don't come into a psychiatrist's office. Why should they? They feel great. As one hyperthymic multimillionaire businessman told me, "I never get down or depressed. Once in a while, however, I lose my optimism." Most of the time, that's as bad as it gets for hyperthymics. When they do fall, they are called moody people by their family and friends and ideally diagnosed as cyclothymic by their psychiatrists.

Looking back through the distorting lens of their depression, people tend to diminish the importance of their earlier productive periods or even deny that they've ever experienced them at all. That is one reason I like new patients to bring along a close friend or family member; the friend or relative may remember the subtle highs of the past. The graduate student who's always been at the top of her class; the management consultant who lectures around the world; the entrepreneur who has made millions, lost them, and made them again; the scriptwriter who, against all odds, has succeeded in what is a cutthroat occupation: these are not people with only ordinary accom- plishments, no matter how the patients now paint themselves. These are energetic, hyperthymic normals or—if their mood also has a down phase— cyclothymic people. These are the best candidates for Prozac transformation.

If I were to treat these primarily normal people using the mood scale at the end of this book, the diagnosis of hyperthymia or cyclothymia would be made.

What do patients and psychiatrists mean by a normal mood?

The expression "normal mood" is basically an artificial construct. In reality, most people experience mild and transient moodswings. Anyone can feel more down than usual or more up than usual for a few hours or several days; those mild mood fluctuations are part of what we mean by normal. But when the person is always revved up or always down in the dumps, when these up or down feelings become so strong that they go beyond the usual baseline range, psychiatrists begin to consider the mood pathological even if the patient does not.

Patients are likely to define the word normal in individual ways that entirely depend on their personal history. For people with a life-time history of minimal depression, normal *is* for them slightly depressed. To psychiatrists seeing these patients and comparing them with hundreds of other people in the general population, these patients are clearly more depressed than the cultural norm and would be diagnosed as such. These people might be considered hypothymic; their mood is at the bottom of normal or slightly below.

Similarly, hyperthymics who have been energetic, driving, and productive all their lives usually see this as their normal mood. However, experts in mood disorders know that these people are more energetic and active than are most people in the population. These people lead lives at the top of normal or slightly beyond—although they describe themselves as "normal."

Are people who are prone to hyperthymia, hypomania, or cyclothymia considered manic or manic depressive?

Yes, in a sense, since manic depression is a spectrum disease. They fall somewhere on what has been called the soft bipolar continuum. However, their symptoms are less extreme than those of manic depression, and cyclothymic episodes are much shorter in duration.

Does depression (unipolar) ever become manic depression (bipolar)?

Every psychiatrist needs to be aware that a not-so-small percentage of people who seem to be unipolar eventually blossom into bipolarity. This is less rare than one might expect. After following a group of patients at the University of Tennessee Mood Clinic for a period of several years, Dr. Hagop S. Akiskal and his colleagues found that 14% of the patients originally considered "neurotic depressives"—the old term for those afflicted with dysthymia—developed hypomania, and an additional 4% became manic; a total of 18% of the seemingly unipolar patients became bipolar. No wonder so many patients are misdiagnosed. The disease spectrum itself changes shape, and psychiatrists often fail to be good historians or medical detectives. They miss the mild highs, and as a result the patient is misdiagnosed as unipolar depressive, either major or dysthymic, or as having a personality disorder with subclinical depressive symptoms.

How do these bipolar depressed patients react to the older standard antidepressants?

Often quite well. Over the past three decades, I've seen many dramatic responses, both with lithium alone and with lithium combined with the standard antidepressants. But even though people may feel more even-tempered and energetic with older antidepressants, symptoms such as constipation, blurred vision, and weight gain can be very bothersome; and they are all the more unbearable for people whose depression wasn't that bad. The MAOIs present the additional difficulty of prohibiting tyramine-containing substances such as cheese, Chianti wine, chocolates, and other foods and some over-the-counter medications.

In the vast majority of people, the side effects of Prozac are extremely mild or nonexistent.

Do dramatic Prozac responses occur in lifetime chronic depressives without an obvious personal or family history of ups and downs?

Maybe. I'm sure it must happen from time to time. But I have rarely seen it.

Don't misunderstand: many people who are chronic major or minor depressives, so-called dysthymics, can benefit enormously from Prozac or other antidepressants. At least 65% of the time, medication can relieve their depression. These patients may not feel reborn but they will feel markedly better than before and function much better; in short, they will feel "normal."

How does Prozac affect subclinical depression?

With the help of Prozac or other antidepressants, people can come out of the subclinical depressions hidden within personality disorders and feel better than they've ever felt before. This is particularly possible for patients who are given Prozac or other SSRIs, since the side effects are much milder than those associated with the traditional tricyclics and MAOIs. Like Prozac and the other SSRIs, the TCAs and MAOIs may also quickly eliminate the symptoms of depression. But the typical side effects of dry mouth, constipation, blurred vision, and weight gain are troublesome. With Prozac, the worst side effects—temporary nausea, insomnia for two to three days, or a jittery feeling—are temporary, and most patients find that their painful symptoms disappear in one to two weeks. When that happens, the distinctions between before and after become so crystal-clear that these people may claim to feel better than they've ever felt in their lives–"better than normal," thanks to the antidepressant's effects on the hidden depressive symptoms. The therapist may call this a complex personality transformation, but to me it's much simpler. It has nothing to do with defense mechanisms, transference, or interpretation of dreams; it's the antidepressant working effectively and biochemically on the serotonergic system at the synapses of the brain, a process which can alter symptoms of the unrecognized subclinical depression.

What is a personality disorder? Is Prozac effective in treating or changing it?

An individual with a personality disorder is someone who responds to internal or external stress with thoughts, perceptions, or patterns of behavior so inflexible, extreme, and beyond the normal range that the person's level of functioning is seriously impaired. The term is not used to describe single episodes of inappropriate behavior or ideas. Rather, it refers to long-term patterns of thought or behavior.

The *DSM-IV* divides personality disorders into three groups. Paranoid, schizophrenic, and schizotypal disorders compromise Cluster A. Cluster B, the so-called dramatic, emotional, or erratic cluster, includes antisocial, borderline, histrionic, and narcissistic disorders. Cluster C, known as the anxious or fearful cluster, includes avoidant, dependent, passive-aggressive, and obsessive compulsive disorders.

According to a number of psychiatrists, Prozac and other SSRI antidepressants have enabled patients with personality disorders to function normally—in many cases for the first time in their lives. For instance, in borderline personality disorders treated with Prozac, preliminary data indicate significant improvement in impulse control, suicidal and agressive behavior, and depression.

Personality disorder diagnoses frequently overlap and coexist with other conditions including major depression, dysthymia, panic disorder, bulimia, alcoholism, and drug abuse, some of which may respond to Prozac and other SSRIs, presumably due to their ability to increase the synaptic level of serotonin in the brain.

Is it justified to give Prozac to anyone who enters a physician's office and asks for it for a personality change?

In my opinion, no—unless a thorough psychiatric evaluation reveals a previously undiagnosed condition, usually one of the depressive disorders, which the scientific literature the FDA and the community of psychiatrists support as responsive to Prozac. Subclinical depression may be underdiagnosed and overlooked, resulting in its misdiagnosis as a personality disorder only, when in fact its one or two symptoms are hidden. This in my mind often justifies a trial of Prozac, and the patient usually responds well, particularly when the psychotherapy the patient is undergoing is stalemated and does not seem to be progressing.

Does Prozac remove the "static" that is making me think in a fuzzy way? Does it give me new brain power?

Prozac won't make anyone smarter or more knowledgeable. But it can clear up the fuzziness that depressed patients complain about and speed up the thinking process. This is a result of eliminating depression. People suffering from major depression or from low-grade dysthymic depression can't concentrate; their thinking and speech are often slowed down; their memory may be slightly impaired; they may feel bewildered by simple decisions. Not surprisingly, they often do poorly at work and in school. This can be reversed.

By relieving the depression, Prozac can clear away the fuzziness. The memory improves. Patients can focus again. Words and ideas flow more readily. Because they feel more hopeful and less anxious, they can make decisions more forcefully. In this sense, Prozac can give renewed thinking power.

Can Prozac be prescribed for low self-esteem?

Although not approved by the FDA for low self-esteem only, Prozac has been approved for major depression. It and minor depression (dysthymia) usually include a common symptom of low self-esteem. Thus, a detailed history should probe for other symptoms of depression or subclinical depression. If either is detected, I would try Prozac or another antidepressant drug.

Can Prozac make people less sensitive to rejection?

A trivial remark or a minor slight, however unintended, can feel like a major blow to people who are temporarily suffering from depression. For others, sensitivity to rejection (real or imagined) can seem to be a lifelong personality trait, virtually inborn, although it does not have to be categorized as an inevitable part of personality.

Sensitivity to rejection, as proposed by Donald F. Klein, can also be one of the symptoms that characterize atypical depression, along with overeating, oversleeping, and reactivity to the environment. By alleviating the overall atypical depressive syndrome, Prozac can reduce the exquisite sensitivity that causes patients to feel so easily hurt, rejected or snubbed. MAOI antidepressants have this same property, but because their side effects are more intrusive, Prozac may be the better solution for a patient who is easily hurt and becomes depressed each time.

Has Prozac been successfully used to treat social phobia?

Social phobia is an anxiety disorder marked by a strong, persistent fear of certain social situations—especially those involving strangers or those in which the person expects scrutiny (such as public speaking). The apprehension and the fear of embarrassment or humiliation are so great that people who suffer from social phobia typically avoid the dreaded situations completely. Although in all other aspects of living they may function quite normally, they often have excuses for not participating in social situations and they may deny that their fear exists. They have been treated successfully with TCAs as well as MAOIs in the past. Recent reports indicate that Prozac has also been used successfully to treat social phobia. In my practice, I have seen a number of social phobics dramatically improve on Prozac as well as MAOIs.

Can Prozac take away the feeling that I am ugly?

This sensation, also known by its official name, *dysmorphic somatoform disorder*, affects more people than one might imagine. Little research has been done on it, but one study reported ten cases in which patients who had a pathological feeling of ugliness were treated successfully with Prozac.

It is also a common element of depression—especially among women. "When you're depressed, you don't think you're pretty. None of your good attributes seem to be real," comments a young bipolar patient of mine. After she made an impressive turnaround on a combination of lithium and Prozac, that feeling disappeared. "To me, it's a remarkable thing now just to be able to look at myself, just to say, Gee, I'm really attractive," she says. "It's a very strange thing, because that good feeling could have been there before; I just don't feel it when I'm depressed. The depression robs me of any objectivity or any belief that I am good or that there is anything good about me. Depression was like a smokescreen in front of me or a veil that lifted after I took Prozac with lithium."

Can Prozac decrease suspiciousness in otherwise normal people?

Considerable evidence suggests that it can. Although the family (and even the psychiatrist) may see the suspicious character trait as the only bothersome symptom, the suspiciousness may be masking an unrecognized depression. In these cases, Prozac alleviates the underlying clinical or subclinical depression, which in turn causes the patient to feel less suspicious or paranoid. Phobias and feelings of panic that accompany depression usually clear up as well, once the depressed symptoms are alleviated.

Does Prozac affect creativity?

Certainly depression does. The tendency toward depression and manic depression seems to be common in creative people, but when they are in the grip of the beast itself, creativity seems to wither or die. For instance, the nineteenth-century composer Robert Schumann, a manic-depressive who made two failed suicide attempts and finally starved himself to death in an insane asylum at the age of 46, produced dozens of compositions yearly during his periods of hypomania—and little or nothing in the years of his darkest depressions. Many writers, musicians, and painters have complained to me that when they are depressed, they feel unable to write, to compose, to play their musical instrument, or to pick up their brushes to paint.

Prozac can alleviate this block by eliminating the depression and lifting the mood, thereby igniting the creative spark.

It cannot, however, make a creative artist out of a person who has never been creative—unless a depression has somehow hidden or blocked the creativity.

In some patients, Prozac brings the individual out of a depression into a revved-up, slightly hypomanic state. Patients claim that in that state they work faster and focus better. The creativity may be unchanged, but the productivity zooms. Consider Vincent van Gogh. During periods he described as "furies of painting," van Gogh stopped eating and sleeping for days at a time and was incredibly productive. In 1888, he painted two hundred canvases in two months. But although these manic highs were productive and creative, they were also dangerously unstable. Sometimes, he calmed down and had periods of lucidity and calm (a serenity reflected in the style of the paintings he made at these times); but too often, the productive high led inexorably to psychotic periods of mania, paranoia, and violence. In addition to being repeatedly hospitalized, van Gogh attacked his friend Gauguin with a razor, cut off his own ear, threatened to shoot his friend Dr. Gachet, and ultimately, at the age of 37, took his own life.

What is the relationship between manic-depressive illness and creativity?

In the more than forty years since the discovery and later the widespread use of lithium for manic depression, scientific and clinical case studies have been accumulating rapidly, showing a high rate of severe mood disorders and suicides among artists, composers, sculptors, and writers. Researchers at the University of Kentucky Medical Center reviewed the lives of over a thousand accomplished people in a variety of fields, including Henri Matisse, Aldous Huxley, and Albert Einstein. 17% of the actors and 13% of the poets were manic-depressives—but only about 1% of the scientists. Other studies have found that manic depression and major depression are as much as ten to thirty times more frequent among noted artists than among the population as a whole.

A study matching thirty members of the Iowa Writers' Workshop with thirty nonwriters revealed that 80% of the writers—but only 30% of the nonwriters—reported at least one episode of depression or manic depression (30% of the writers but only 6% of the controls, were alcoholic). In addition, the parents and siblings of the writers were significantly more creative and more prone to highs and lows than the relatives of the nonwriters. For instance, 20% of the writers' brothers and sisters, but only 3% of the siblings of the control population, had a mood disorder; 14% of the writers' siblings had experienced major depression, versus 3% of the control siblings.

This data strongly suggests a genetic link between mania, depression, and artistic creativity.

Is Prozac overprescribed?

Yes. But the many people who have heard remarkable stories about Prozac's effects on mood, personality, and behavior have requested Prozac—and not just from their psychiatrists. They have asked their general physicians, their surgeons, even their dermatologists and dentists to give them Prozac, and many times these doctors have wrongly complied, giving it to patients for whom it is not justified. Nevertheless, even while Prozac is incorrectly and even overprescribed for some people, it is a documented fact that 50% of all depressed people go totally undiagnosed and untreated. This figure amounts to millions. Many of these could benefit from Prozac and other antidepressant drugs.

In my opinion, patients who do not suffer from one of the depressive disorder spectrum diagnoses (these include major depression, dysthymia, and subclinical depression as well as many of the personality disorders with at least one or two of the required symptoms of major depression—the so-called formes fruste type) or obsessive-compulsive disorder, should be treated with Prozac only with great caution, because scientific evidence has not been sufficient to gain FDA approval. If Prozac is being prescribed for any illness other than major depression and OCD, it should be considered experimental by the patient and physician, and the patient should be so informed. Caution should be observed.

• 9 •

Who Should Take Prozac?
Who Should Have Therapy?

Who should take Prozac?

Prozac is especially helpful for patients with major depression, dysthymia (the milder version of major depression), and obsessive-compulsive disorder, as well as for patients who lack energy, feel listless, and chronically function below par, symptoms typically seen in subclinical depression. In addition, psychiatrists who have read individual claims of Prozac's usefulness in treating bulimia and other disorders can probably feel safe prescribing Prozac to individual patients with these symptoms.

However, the FDA has not completed its evaluations, and in the meantime, Prozac has not yet been approved for anything other than major depression and obsessive-compulsive disorder. Despite its popularity, Prozac should be prescribed with care and not simply handed out to anyone who wants it.

What are the different phases in the treatment of depression?

Depression experts and psychopharmacologists have conceptualized the treatment of depression into three parts: the acute phase, the continuation phase, and the maintenance phase.

The *acute phase* of treatment begins when the patient appears in the doctor's office showing signs or complaining of symptoms of depression. At this point, the immediate goal is to alleviate the symptoms as quickly as possible. This might mean medication, some form of psychotherapy, or a combination of the two.

The *continuation or middle phase* of treatment begins once the patient has responded to treatment. Too frequently, both the patient and the physician, believing that an improvement of symptoms indicates that the depression has been defeated, discontinue the medication. This is a mistake. Although the depression may have retreated, often it has not yet been conquered. It is simply in remission. If the patient is taken off medication too soon, the depression may attack again. Even with medication, relapses are common, which is why it is important to continue treatment during this phase. To prevent a relapse after the symptoms have disappeared, one study found that patients need to continue taking medication for four or five months. My clinical experience backs this up.

During the third or *maintenance phase* of treatment, the object is to prevent another acute episode of depression. The way to do this is by maintaining the medication for as long as several years—or a lifetime. Patients often don't want to do this, sometimes because they just don't like the idea of taking drugs and they feel that they are "cured." Yet the unfortunate fact is that for most people, depression is not a once-in-a-lifetime event. More than 50% of patients suffering from a first bout of major depression will have it again at some point, and 80% to 90% of patients having a second episode will go on to experience a third. With disorders such as major depression, preventive medicine *means* long-term maintenance medication.

Emerging evidence also suggests that many depressed patients do better if medication is combined with three or four months of individual psychotherapy, cognitive therapy, or behavioral therapy. When the therapy comes to an end, however, the medication should continue if the depression is recurrent.

What is cognitive therapy?

Cognitive therapy is a short-term structured form of psychotherapy based on the idea that the way a patient perceives the world determines behavior. The tendency to see oneself, the world about one, and the future in a negative way often leads to depression, according to this school of thought. Treatment is aimed at altering these cognitive misperceptions by helping patients gather evidence to counteract this distorted view.

What is behavioral therapy?

Behavioral therapy is a form of psychotherapy that aims to inhibit or extinguish "learned" neurotic responses. Techniques include assertiveness training, biofeedback, aversive therapy, conditioning, contract therapy, flooding, and desensitization. There are a limited number of reports that certain illnesses responsive to Prozac, including OCD and phobias, are more effectively treated with the combination of behavioral therapy and Prozac or older antidepressants than with medication alone.

What other forms of therapy are effective for the treatment of depression?

Interpersonal Psychotherapy (IPT) is a three-part, time-limited therapy specifically designed to help alleviate major depression. During the first one to three sessions, the psychotherapist takes a psychiatric history and an interpersonal inventory that focuses on the patient's psychosocial problems. The middle phase of IPT focuses on the problems of the present (rather than the past) through a series of strategies designed to help the patient cope with grief, interpersonal conflicts, role transitions, and inadequate social skills. During the final phase, the therapist helps the patient learn to recognize and cope with symptoms of depression that might appear in the future.

Various studies have shown that IPT is an effective therapy for some forms of depression even without drugs. This is important because there are many instances in which depressed patients cannot take drugs. Some people are simply not responsive to drugs, some experience uncomfortable or even dangerous side effects, and some have other medical conditions that make taking the drug problematic (pregnancy might be one such condition). However, the best results, especially during the acute phase of major depression, came from the combination of cognitive therapy or IPT with an antidepressant medication.

Is depression inherited?

The predisposition to depression definitely runs in families. Studies have shown that the "first-degree" relatives—parents, children, and siblings—of depressives are two or three times more likely to become depressed than the relatives of a normal control group.

The genetic link is particularly strong among manic-depressives, approximately 50% of whom have at least one parent afflicted with major depression or another mood disorder. Among children with one bipolar parent, 27% will have a mood disorder; when both parents are bipolar, the chances jump to 50% to 75%.

The importance of this cannot be underestimated for both the patients and their families. Thousands of parents are beginning to understand that it was not their faulty parenting that caused the sadly chaotic or wasted lives of their children with mood disorders. The cause is principally biological and genetic (although environment and events certainly can precipitate depression in those with the genetic tendency). As we gain more understanding about manic and depressive illness, both bipolar and unipolar, and as researchers find more effective treatments, guilt is being lifted from these families. While depression is for the most part an inherited disease, it is also easily treatable.

Over the past thirty years, enormous strides have been made in the diagnosis and treatment of mood disorders. New findings on the genetics of depression, a biological test for depression (the dexamethasone test), and precise blood measurements of lithium and antidepressant medications are now a reality. In my private practice, these tests and services are available on the premises.

Just as people in the past suffered and died from physical ailments now easily cured or prevented by medication, at least eleven million people in the United States today suffer from depressive disorders that are equally controllable. They wake up filled with dread, walk down the street wondering if they should step in front of a truck, and feel so unmotivated that sometimes they can't even force themselves to take a shower or pick up the telephone. But these mood disorders don't have to ruin people's lives. With Prozac, lithium, and other drugs, new and old, they can be controlled.

Are there other biological factors?

The most well-known biological factor is the mysterious, incontrovertible fact that women are at least twice as likely as men to become depressed.

On the other hand, manic depression strikes men and women equally.

What about ordinary life events? Don't they make a difference?

Of course they do. One specific event known to strengthen the likelihood of major depression in adulthood is the death of a parent, particularly before a child reaches the age of 11. Normal grief that follows the death of a spouse can trigger a major depression, especially when there is genetic vulnerability.

Nonetheless, a family history of affective disorders is a stronger predictor of depression than the stress associated with life events.

Do young people suffer from the same side effects of Prozac as adults?

Not entirely. In large clinical trials of Prozac, the most commonly felt side effects in adults were nausea (21.2%) and headache (20.3%), while in an open study of a small group of young people, the most frequent side effects were restlessness (27%) and sweating (20%). Drowsiness, dry mouth, tremor, and thinning hair also showed up more frequently in the young people than in adults. Compared to other antidepressants, these side effects were minimal both in young people and in adults.

Another unwanted, sometimes severe, reaction that appears more frequently among young people is mania. A published study described five adolescent girls, all with family histories riddled with major depression and suicide, who developed mania while taking Prozac. Considering the surprising fact that young people who experience serious major depression before the age of 18 almost invariably become bipolar, it is imperative to watch carefully for the development of these symptoms.

The need still exists for carefully controlled clinical studies comparing the responses of children and adolescents to Prozac and other standard drugs. In the meantime, youngsters taking Prozac should be observed closely and frequently by their families, and any side effects should be immediately reported to the psychiatrist.

What are the risk factors that might predispose adolescents to becoming manic after treatment with Prozac?

Risk factors that might lead to possible mania among adolescents taking Prozac are:

- a diagnosis of bipolar disorder
- a family history of affective disorders, and especially of bipolar disorders
- unstable moods of a milder degree
- major depression with psychotic features
- attention deficit hyperactivity disorder.

Can Prozac be safely used by elderly people who are depressed?

This is an important question, because depression hits the elderly hard. Depression is four times more common among the elderly than in the general population, and the suicide rate for people over 65 is fifteen times greater than that of the overall population.

John P. Feighner and his International Clinical Research (ICR) team investigated Prozac's effects on the elderly, using at least two methodologies: double blind studies, in which some patients were given Prozac and some patients received tricyclic antidepressants, but neither patients nor researchers knew who got what, and open studies, which lack a control group. Both types of studies indicate that Prozac relieves the symptoms of depression as effectively as other antidepressants in geriatric patients. But patients taking Prozac complained less frequently of dry mouth, constipation, and drowsiness. As a result, they were much less likely to stop taking the drug due to adverse effects. Some 55% to 56.8% of the patients on tricyclic antidepressants dropped out of various studies, whereas 45% to 47.1% of the Prozac patients discontinued.

Prozac lacks adverse cardiovascular effects, compared to the tricyclic drugs, and is much less dangerous in overdose. Thus, most psychopharmacologists prefer Prozac as an antidepressant in the elderly.

Prescribing physicians should consider giving elderly patients lower dosages, especially when the patient has physical problems or is on a variety of other medications.

When should a patient take Prozac as opposed to another antidepressant?

Prozac is a particularly beneficial treatment for:

- patients who are sensitive to side effects of medications in general, and especially the side effects of tricyclic antidepressants and MAOIs

- patients who dislike taking pills, since Prozac can be taken as one pill a day or in liquid form rather than the three to six capsules a day often needed with the tricyclics and MAOIs

- patients who have tried to overdose on other antidepressant drugs

- patients with cardiovascular disease, since Prozac's effects on blood pressure and the electrocardiogram appear to be minimal (however, patients with unstable heart disease and recent myocardial infarction were not included in early studies).

Will Prozac turn me into a bubbly energetic extrovert?

Depression makes people more introverted, isolated, less energetic, and withdrawn in the way they express their emotions—the precise opposite of bubbly. Prozac can help to lift that depression, with the result that the patient becomes energetic, extroverted, and more positive.

But even Prozac cannot turn a unipolar depressive into a cheerleader or a talk show host—unless the manic predisposition is already there. When it is, in however latent a form, transformations such as those described in Peter Kramer's provocative book *Listening to Prozac* can and do take place. Prozac in that case does seem to have the ability to turn whining nitpickers into optimists, to allow longtime depressives to wake up looking forward to the day, and to give previously depressed people the wherewithal to make important changes in their lives. A limited number of psychiatrists have reported seeing major metamorphoses in these patients—more so than with other antidepressants, even though those medications also produced striking changes.

Still, the issue is a fuzzy one, because the evidence is based more on patient perception and physician perspicacity than on anything measurable with standard diagnostic tools. This question has yet to be studied in a scientific way. I've given my explanation in Chapter 8 for the up to 10% of patients who undergo transformation with Prozac. I believe these people already had a mild tendency to experience elevated moods. With Prozac, they were finally able to achieve consistently this high level of functioning.

Should Prozac be used instead of psychotherapy or in addition to it?

The relationship of medication to psychotherapy has been debated endlessly. Although it would be difficult to find a psychoanalytically trained psychiatrist who never prescribes medication or a psychopharmacologist who never recommends therapy, it is nonetheless true that most psychiatrists fall on one side or the other of this great divide. Either they passionately believe that psychotherapy (or another form of talk therapy) is the preferred treatment, or they believe, as I do, that medication should generally come first.

The issue is particularly important in terms of the treatment of depression. Few would argue the importance of medication for illnesses such as schizophrenia or severe manic depression. But people often feel different about depression, especially if it is mild or moderate. Increasingly few professionals question the necessity of medication in cases of moderate to severe depression. However, there is still a tendency, to blame the victims, to believe that if they will only get themselves together, confront their issues, and deal forthrightly with their fears either in treatment or by themselves, they would feel less depressed—without medication. Medication, in this sense, is seen as a weak second choice to be made only when therapy has failed.

My clinical experiences have led me to some very different conclusions. Certainly there are times when therapy is all that is required, and in those instances it can be very effective, arming patients with much-needed support and hard-won insights and helping them drop destructive old behaviors and substitute constructive new ones.

But often that doesn't happen. Over the course of my career, I've seen far too many patients who, after years of weekly or twice-weekly appointments, are still struggling with depression. And even when the therapy has been declared successful and the depression appears to have exited forever, it is merely dormant, awaiting its biological cue for spontaneous recurrence. In an enormous percentage of patients, depression returns.

It doesn't have to. I believe that for an extraordinarily large number of patients who are now being given psychotherapy alone for various forms of depression, overt or hidden, Prozac or another antidepressant is the treatment of choice and should be given either in conjunction with psychotherapy or instead of it. Ideally, medication should be accompanied by some form of psychotherapy especially in the first three or four months. But if it is necessary to pick either medication or therapy, the choice is clear. Medication can return a depressed patient to a normal emotional state by eliminating symptoms, including the urge to commit suicide. If the patient wants to enter psychotherapy in addition to taking medication, so much the better; a number of studies have now demonstrated that patients recovering from acute episodes of major depression do better when they are receiving both therapy and an antidepressant drug than they do with medication alone.

Does Prozac effectively treat disorders other than depression?

In July 1993, the FDA unanimously approved Prozac as a treatment for obsessive-compulsive disorder, a widespread ailment that affects approximately 5 million Americans.

OCD causes people, virtually against their will, to become obsessed with certain thoughts and to indulge in time-consuming behaviors such as washing their hands repeatedly, checking and rechecking that the doors and windows are locked, counting or touching compulsively, being inordinately concerned with arranging objects in specific, often symmetrical ways, and many other irrational actions. Although behavioral therapy can be successful on its own, the best treatment is therapy combined with medication.

The three most effective medications used to treat OCD are Anafranil, Prozac, and fluvoxamine, an SSRI recently approved for OCD in the United States.

Is Prozac an effective treatment for anxiety?

Yes—if the anxiety is secondary to depression, as it often is. Evidence clearly suggests that Prozac and the other SSRIs are as effective as tricyclic antidepressants in decreasing the anxiety felt by depressed patients. It is not approved for primary anxiety disorders, which are best treated with a combination of tranquilizers and psychotherapy.

For a small percentage of patients, Prozac can increase anxiety. In clinical tests, 9.4% of the patients reported feeling anxiety as a side effect, and 14.9% complained of nervousness.

Is Prozac an effective treatment for panic attacks and agoraphobia?

Yes, it is. Prozac has a powerful effect on the frightening bursts of anxiety and rising waves of panic that characterize panic disorder, the symptoms of which include shortness of breath, dizziness, rapid heartbeat, sweaty palms, trembling, choking, chest pain, and fear of going crazy, passing out, or dying. In one study, nineteen out of twenty-five patients who were treated with Prozac for panic disorder and, in some cases, agoraphobia, showed moderate to remarkable improvement in their symptoms. Treatment was most effective when it started at the low level of 5 mg a day.

It is likely that Prozac and other medications, by alleviating panic attacks, can also cause a decrease in the symptoms of agoraphobia, the debilitating fear of open spaces, including going into crowded streets and department stores, that often results in patients becoming completely housebound, sometimes for years on end.

Behavioral therapy, typically including exercises aimed at desensitizing the patient to frightening stimuli, also plays an important role in the treatment of both panic disorder and agoraphobia. For my patients with panic disorder, agoraphobia, or social phobia, I use a combination of an antidepressant and behavioral therapy.

Is Prozac an effective treatment for post-traumatic stress disorder (PTSD)?

Once known as shell shock, post-traumatic stress disorder afflicts the survivors of dire catastrophes such as childhood abuse, wartime battles, confinement in concentration camps, assault, rape, being in a fire, or seeing another person killed. People suffering from this syndrome feel numbed, irritable, anxious, and depressed, in part because the memory of the trauma plays over and over in their mind and is often so vivid that it may feel real for years after the event. Several reports have indicated that patients treated with Prozac show a lessening of PTSD symptoms.

In patients with PTSD, I consider psychotherapy the major treatment modality. Medications, while helpful, are secondary.

Is Prozac effective in treating eating disorders such as bulimia?

Bulimia nervosa, with its terrible pattern of compulsive eating binges, self-induced vomiting, laxative and diuretic abuse, and anything else its sufferers can think of to control their weight, affects between 1.3% and 10.1% of American women. Although older antidepressants, especially the MAOIs, have been shown to help, side effects frequently have presented problems, in part because they often include weight gain, which bulimics fear to an alarming degree. Prozac does not usually have that unwanted effect. In an eight-week test involving close to four hundred women who daily were randomly given 20 mg of Prozac, 60 mg of Prozac, or a placebo, the medication reduced eating binges in up to 63% of the responders and episodes of vomiting in up to 57%. In this study, the larger dose proved more effective than the smaller dose.

Psychotherapy or behavioral therapy in combination with medication has proven to be the most effective treatment for bulimia.

Is Prozac useful with any other disorders?

Preliminary studies of a small number of patients diagnosed with borderline personality disorder and schizophrenia have reported definite improvement with Prozac. Although much research still needs to be done, the evidence so far is encouraging. For instance, in a ten-week study of eight treatment-resistant chronic schizophrenics, every one showed improvement with Prozac. They became less aggressive, more socially interactive, and more involved in hospital programs. One of them was even discharged.

Substance abuse—whether it is alcohol, cocaine, or other addictive drugs—is most effectively treated with Alcoholics Anonymous, self-help groups, and group therapies. Patients with depressive symptoms should be evaluated for concomitant use of antidepressants.

What do I do if my depression has not been relieved by Prozac, Zoloft, Paxil, or Wellbutrin, as well as the typical older TCAs and MAOIs?

Many psychiatrists recommend augmentation treatment by adding lithium or a thyroid hormone, Cytomel. Oftentimes the addition of one or both of these drugs to the antidepressant boosts the patient out of depression. Both drugs are considered step-up treatments. However, if the psychopharmacological approach does not work, consider psychotherapy.

In extreme cases, in which the patient is suicidal, losing weight, or totally unresponsive to any of the above medication, electroconvulsive therapy has proved very useful. Despite the negative associations some people have about ECT, it is a proven therapy that can rapidly and effectively treat serious depression.

Finally, patients who are treatment resistant to all medications on the market may wish to consider participating in a free clinical research trial on a new antidepressant compound that is being evaluated at a number of universities and clinical research centers throughout the country *(see Chapter 2 for more information on this topic).*

• 10 •

The Challenge to Prozac:
Drugs Present and Future

Although Prozac is a remarkable drug that has erased the symptoms of depression in millions of people, it doesn't work for everyone. As with every other antidepressant, Prozac fails to eliminate depression in about one third of the people who take it. Fortunately, several new drugs that have been recently approved by the FDA and released to the public offer exciting treatment possibilities for patients who have not responded to other medications. These newly developed antidepressants present a challenge to Prozac. Among them are:

- Zoloft (sertraline), launched in 1991, is an selective serotonin re-uptake inhibitor (SSRI) with the same mild side effect profile as Prozac as well as the same biochemical action. The main difference is that Zoloft has a much shorter half-life, twenty-six hours, which means that it is discharged from the body more quickly than Prozac. The efficacy of the two drugs appears equal, and Zoloft is also equal in antidepressant potency to the older tricyclics and MAOIs. Like Prozac, Zoloft can produce hypomania in genetically susceptible people.

- Paxil (paroxetine), launched in 1993, is another SSRI that is similar to Prozac in side effect profile and antidepressant potency. It has a half-life of twenty-one hours.

- Effexor (venlafaxine), an FDA-approved drug that appears to be equal in potency to Prozac and the other SSRIs, has a similarly mild side effect profile, an onset of action that may be somewhat faster, but a different molecular structure. Like the SSRIs, Effexor blocks the uptake of serotonin, and like the older antidepressants, it blocks the uptake of norepinephrine, thereby increasing the levels of these two neurotransmitter hormones in the brain. By acting on both neurotransmitters and thus, presumably, attacking depression that is caused not only by serotonin deficiency but also by norepinephrine deficiency, Effexor may treat a broader range of depressive disorders than the SSRIs. A single unconfirmed study on inpatient depressives in France suggests that Effexor may be more effective than Prozac in treating this group of severely depressed patients. Effexor is being marketed as an antidepressant drug that is effective in chronic- or treatment-resistant depressions as well as in treating people for whom the SSRIs have not worked. Effexor has been tested successfully over the past five to seven years both in Europe and in the United States.

- Luvox (fluvoxamine) is a fourth SSRI that has been approved by the FDA for obsessive compulsive disorder. Its efficacy in OCD appears to equal that of Prozac and Anafranil. Although it has not yet gained FDA approval as a treatment for depression in the United States, it has been used as an antidepressant for several years in Europe and Canada.

- Serzone (nefazadone) is the fifth SSRI to be approved in the United States and is similar to Prozac, Zoloft, and Paxil in its side effect profile, effectiveness, and onset of action. Currently, Serzone is being compared to Zoloft and Prozac for possible differences in side effects found by my research team and a number of other researchers throughout the United States. Several years will be needed to produce and analyze this data, but in the meantime Serzone will be appearing on the market and competing with the other medications.

In addition to these new drugs, all of which are presently in use, there are at least ten to fifteen potential antidepressants in various stages of development worldwide. These include Citalopram (an SSRI), the so-called "gentle" antidepressants, including brofaromine, Aurorix (moclobemide), and Humeril (toloxotone), and the antidepressants rolipram, dexfenfluramine, ritanserin, and milnacipran. Some of these are already being marketed in Europe and all of them are currently undergoing trials in the United States.

What research is currently being undertaken to develop new antidepressant treatments?

Hundreds of laboratories, outpatient clinics, and university inpatient units around the world are searching for the causes of depression and manic depression, as well as developing new treatments. Biochemical, genetic, and behavioral research is being conducted, and many research centers both public and private are actively exploring new pharmacologic treatments in the expectation that they can develop new and better drugs that work faster, are safer and more effective, and have fewer side effects.

Much progress has been made. New drugs not yet on the market are being tested. There is good reason to believe that antidepressants even more effective that Prozac will eventually be developed. Since the 1970s, lithium has brought unimagined help to manic depressives. Now Prozac and other newly developed antidepressant compounds are offering relief from forms of depression that the older antidepressants failed to eliminate. New drugs being tested today should increase the number of patients who, though they may currently feel marooned on a desolate island or isolated beneath a dark cloud that never lifts, can in the near future look forward to a better, happier, more productive life that is symptom-free.

How do I get to be chosen for a clinical trial?

Free drug trials are advertised on radio and television and in the newspapers. Upon telephoning the investigator, a potential participant in one of these trials would undergo a ten-minute screening interview on the phone, during which the new drug, the nature of the study, and the possibility of being assigned to a placebo would be explained, along with the rights of patients who volunteer, including the right to discontinue the drug at any time. If the screening interview looks promising, the patient is asked to come in for a more detailed psychiatric interview. Thereafter, a medical exam, including an EKG, is performed to see if the patient is truly eligible. If the patient meets the criteria, he or she is asked to sign a one- or two-page informed consent document about the study.

Clinical drug studies generally fall into three categories. In phase I studies, patients in the hospital are treated with drugs in their earliest state of clinical development to determine dosages and safety. In phase II studies, both hospitalized patients and outpatients are given low, medium, or high doses to check for efficacy, tolerance, and side effects. In phase III studies, investigators usually compare the new drug to a placebo and to one or two other standard drugs that have been marketed for several years. Large numbers of outpatients in eight to ten centers throughout the country participate thereafter in a six- to eight-week trial. Most new drug studies go through these final phases of development prior to approval by the FDA for marketing. In phase IV, drug studies take place after marketing in order to investigate the medication's potential usefulness with diseases other than the initial illness for which the FDA gave its approval. The people who participate in these antidepressant trials may include treatment-resistant patients who have tried other antidepressants, including tricyclics, MAOIs, and SSRIs, all without success. For them a new drug trial is the court of last appeal. The lack of cost to the participants and the extraordinary attention they receive from highly qualified doctors and nurses are major factors in the patient's motivation to participate.

What is the main purpose of the psychotropic drug development?

These is a continuous quest in all areas of medicine to develop new drugs with more specific mechanisms that those that are currently available. Psychotropic drugs presently available for treatment of mood disorders, although safe and effective, pose certain problems to many individuals in the form of adverse effects or poor response. Scientists make it their goal to improve upon medication by developing and testing new compounds with the hope of producing a marketable compound far superior to those that have been available to the general public. Prozac, which was not marketed for a full fifteen years after it was developed in 1972, is a successful example of this lengthy process.

What is clinical drug research?

Once a compound has been developed and all pre-clinical work is complete, inlcuding animal pharmacology and toxicology testing, a pharmaceutical company must be granted permission by the Food and Drug Administration to move into clinical trials. At this point, an investigational medication is administered for the first time to a small number of medically healthy, hospitalized volunteers and rigorously evaluated for its safety. Physicians such as myself who conduct clinical drug trials agree to oversee and evaluate the use of an investigational medication. They are responsible for the selection of patients according to the research protocol developed by the pharmaceutical company and approved by an investigational review board (IRB), which guarantees to the patient his or her human rights in participating (including dropping out if desired). Regulations are set forth by the FDA. The FDA has developed a guideline entitled *General Considerations for the Clinical Evaluation of Drugs* along with several more specific documents such as *Guidelines for the Clinical Evaluation of Antidepressant Drugs*.

Are there risks to a patient who participates in a clinical research study?

With any medication, standard marketed drugs or investigational drugs, there is always some risk of adverse side effects. For this reason, patients entered into psychotropic research trials are required to be in excellent health and in a certain age range. (Females of child-bearing potential may not participate.) Numerous safety evaluations are completed and the results are reviewed by a highly qualified medical team prior to dispensing the medication. Physical examinations, electrocardiograms, blood work, and a detailed medical and psychiatric history are all required along with the patient's signed consent. In addition, each patient's progress is monitored very closely by the research team, the pharmaceutical company's clinical team, the investigational review board (IRB), and the FDA.

Possible side effects are explained in advance and patients are able to report these problems any time, night or day. If these side effects pose a risk to the patient, or are too bothersome, discontinuation of medication would be immediately recommended. If during the study, investigators see unexpected adverse effects in their patients, this information is immediately reported to the drug company, which in turn may stop the drug and inform the FDA, if indicated.

All in all, the high degree of monitoring means that the risk is minimal. Once in a while, however, problems do occur. But during the more than twenty years that I have been doing clinical research trials on a large number of CNS (central nervous system) drugs, most of which were eventually marketed, I have seen very few patients who reported serious adverse side effects, and in all cases, once the patient discontinued taking the drug, the side effects subsided.

What is a humanitarian protocol?

Scientific testing is essential for the development of new drugs, but it can sometimes seem heartless to the layman. For instance, many clinical trials for new drugs only last six to eight weeks. Thereafter, no matter how much better a participant might feel, the drug can no longer be obtained until it is fully approved and available on the market. When a patient who has been otherwise unresponsive to all other marketed compounds does extremely well on an investigational new drug, it seems cruel to withdraw the medication. Fortunately, once the testing period is over, a humanitarian protocol is available for a limited number of outpatients taking antidepressant, antianxiety and other psychiatric and medical drugs from pharmaceutical companies testing these compounds. After the initial trial, a patient may report a great improvement of symptoms along with the information that no other drug on or off the market has worked so well as the investigational drug. The patient, through the principal clinical research investigator, may then apply to the drug company with this information, and upon evaluation by the company, the patient may be given the drug to be monitored through the clinical investigator, even though it has not been approved by the FDA for release to the general public.

This is a great humanitarian boon to a limited number of patients who have been chronically depressed for years or suffered other illnesses that can be relieved only by a drug still in a premarketing stage of development. In these instances, the hoped-for improvement the patient found through agreeing to participate in a scientific protocol did not turn out to be temporary. The slight risk the patient took was worth it.

How can you justify the gigantic costs of developing a new antidepressant drug?

Depression is epidemic, affecting more people than virtually any other illness and costing the nation $43.7 billion annually. Only one third of depressed patients seek treatment, yet the reality is that not all of these people are finding the treatment they need—in part because some patients are unresponsive to available medications. The right treatments for them do not exist and are awaiting development. Every time a new drug is developed, hundreds of thousands of people can be successfully treated. Their lives improve. They work more efficiently. (A depressed patient who has received adequate treatment loses half as much time from work as a depressed patient who has not been treated.) A new antidepressant drug can benefit the individual (and the nation) in ways that can be incalculable. As an example, look at Prozac.

• Appendix A •

Dr. Fieve's Self-Rating Mood Scale and Predictors of Prozac Response

From time to time, it is important for persons questioning their own psychological wellbeing to take a look at themselves and to rate their moods and behavior. The reason is that mood affects everything: your personality, your ability to pursue goals and participate in social and professional activities, your creativity, your expression of love and affection, and your capacity to love others and yourself. By using the following chart to rate your mood over a period of weeks, you can become aware of the frequency and depth of your dips into depression (as well as your ascents toward elation) and get an accurate picture of the geography of your own moods. Normal mood fluctuations, as measured against the general population, fall within the area marked by the gray central strip. You will be looking for how often your moods rise above that norm or dip below it, how high or low they go, and how long these moods persist.

On this scale, −5 represents the lowest point of depression, the area from −1 to +1 approximates a normal state (since very few normal people are dead center), and +5 represents the peak of mania. Mark your mood on a daily basis at the same time each morning.

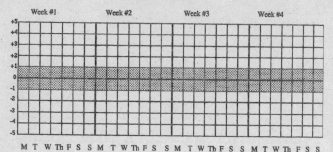

0 **Normal.** No symptoms of depression or manic elation. Functions well in social, professional, and interpersonal areas. Appropriate reactions to daily disappointments and successes.

−1 **Bottom of normal.**

−2 **Hypothymic.** Reasonably well adjusted and functioning adequately, but low-keyed, slightly withdrawn; a follower rather than a leader; smiles infrequently; works efficiently; conscientious; often has obsessive-compulsive or perfectionist personality traits; doing okay.

−3 **Dysthymic.** Mildly depressive mood; low self-confidence; low energy; loss of interest and pleasure; pessimistic; may be a daily mood but if it persists most days for two years, it rates a DSM-IV diagnosis.

−4 **Major Depression.** Depressed mood; loss of interest or pleasure in ordinary activities; loss of energy; disturbed patterns of eating and sleeping; hopelessness; difficulty concentrating or making decisions; suicidal feelings may be present.

−5 **Delusional Psychotic Depression.** Delusions and hallucinations in addition to the symptoms of major depression. Total withdrawal or extreme agitation; a medical emergency.

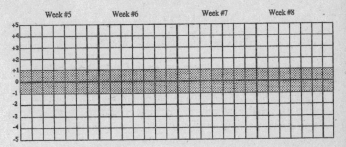

0 **Normal.** No symptoms of depression or of mania. Functions well in social, sexual, professional, and interpersonal areas. Appropriate reactions to daily disappointments and successes.

+1 **Top of normal.**

+2 **Hyperthymic.** Energetic; highly motivated; productive; successful; sociable; sometimes irritable; often a leader in all walks of life; usually well-liked; may need only five to six hours' sleep a night; does not seek therapy.

+3 **Hypomanic.** Predominant mood highly energetic; expansive; elevated; full of ideas and projects; can be angry when crossed and at times irritating; strong sex drive; may compulsively spend money, travel, talk; requires only three to five hours' sleep; poor judgments; risk taking; financial wheeling and dealing may lead to legal consequences.

+4 **Manic.** Elated; overactive; can't stop talking; needs very little or no sleep; highly distractible; racing thoughts; irritable and angry; rage attacks when crossed; extremely poor judgment; depressive features may be present.

+5 **Manic psychosis.** Incoherent; belligerent; out of control; may be violent or paranoid; may have psychotic delusions or hallucinations; high risk taking with painful consequences; depressive features may be present; a medical emergency.

PREDICTORS OF PROZAC RESPONSE

If you and your physician decide that Prozac might benefit you, the following factors should be taken into consideration. In my experience, taking a comprehensive, detailed past and family history should, in at least two-thirds of depressed patients, give a strong indication of how you will respond to the drug.

Fair to Poor Response

- History of a previous depression with poor response to Prozac, other SSRIs, or other antidepressant drugs.
- Diagnosis of chronic, treatment-resistant depression.
- Negative expectations about or fear of Prozac, pill-taking, or psychiatrists. Believes that drugs don't work.
- Poor overall functioning before this depressive episode.
- Achievements: infrequent and accomplished with difficulty.
- No family history of depression, manic depression, or genetic equivalents such as alcoholism, drug abuse, etc.
- No family history of hypomania.
- Poor response of family members to Prozac or other antidepressants. No bipolar III responders.
- Chronic medical conditions, particularly kidney or liver disease, which demand lower doses of Prozac.

Good Response

- History of a previous depression with good response to Prozac, other SSRIs, or other antidepressant drugs.

- Diagnosis of Major Depressive Disorder or dysthymia with no trace of hyperthymic or hypomanic personality.

- Positive expectations about Prozac, pill-taking, or psychiatrists. Believes that drugs probably work.

- Good overall functioning before this depressive episode.

- Average record of achievements.

- Minimal family history of depression, manic depression, or genetic equivalents such as alcoholism, drug abuse, etc.

- Family history of 1 or 2 relatives with hypomania.

- Good response of family members to Prozac or other antidepressants. May include bipolar III responders.

- Medically healthy.

Transformative Response

- History of previous depression with extraordinary, sometimes transforming, response to Prozac, other SSRIs, or other antidepressant drugs.*

- Diagnosis of Major Depressive Disorder or dysthymia with a positive history of hyperthymia or subclinical hypomania.

---

*Caution: Both patient and physician must be aware of the possibility of a manic reaction and consider pretreatment with lithium.

- Very positive expectations about Prozac, pill-taking, or psychiatrists. Unrealistic belief in efficacy of drugs.

- Excellent overall functioning before this depressive episode.

- Outstanding record of achievements.

- Strong family history of depression, manic depression, or genetic equivalents such as alcoholism, drug abuse, etc. Depressed patient must be pretreated with lithium.

- Strong family history of hypomania, possibly on both sides.

- Extraordinary, sometimes manic, response of family members to Prozac or other antidepressants. May include bipolar III responders.*

- Medically healthy.

Glossary

agitated depression an episode of depression characterized by restlessness, insomnia, and loss of appetite.

agoraphobia fear of open spaces or going out in public; literally, fear of the market place. Often preceded by panic attacks, fear of which can keep the sufferer effectively housebound.

alprazolam the generic name for Xanax.

Alzheimer's disease a degenerative, age-related disease of the brain affecting memory and other mental processes.

amantadine the generic name of Symmetrel.

amineptine the generic name for Survector.

amitriptyline the generic name of Elavil, Endep, and other tricyclic antidepressants.

amoxapine the generic name for Asendin.

Anafranil a tricyclic antidepressant also prescribed as an antiobsessional drug. Its generic name is clomipramine.

analgesic a medication used to reduce pain.

antibiotic a medication such as penicillin or streptomycin used to prevent and treat disease by inhibiting the growth of various microorganisms.

antidepressant a medication prescribed for the treatment of depression.

anxiety an uneasy feeling of worry, apprehension, or distress, often about the future. Its physical components include faster heartbeat, disturbed breathing, trembling, and sweating.

anxiety disorders a category of conditions that includes panic disorder, obsessive-compulsive disorder, post-traumatic stress disorder, and various phobias.

Artane an antispasmodic medication used in the treatment of Parkinsonism. Its generic name is trihexyphenidyl.

Asendin a tricyclic antidepressant. Its generic name is amoxapine.

Ativan an antianxiety medication also prescribed for anxiety accompanied by depression. Its generic name is lorazepam.

atypical bipolar II depression a clinical condition in which patients experience periods of major depression and periods of mild or hypomanic elation.

atypical depression an episode of depression in which the patient is reactive to the environment, sensitive to rejection, and tends to gain weight and sleep more than usual. Typical depression, on the other hand, is frequently characterized by loss of weight and difficulty sleeping.

Aventyl a tricyclic antidepressant. Its generic name is nortriptyline.

barbiturate a habit-forming drug used to induce sleep.

behavioral therapy a form of psychotherapy that attempts to change or eliminate certain habitual patterns of behavior.

Benadryl an over-the-counter antihistamine medication often taken for allergies. It is also useful for motion sickness and Parkinsonism.

beta-adrenergic blockers   a medication often used to lower blood pressure.

bipolar depression   a disorder characterized by episodes of both depression and mania or elation.

bipolar I disorder   a clinical condition characterized by episodes of major depression and episodes of mania or elation that are usually severe enough to necessitate hospitalization. Also known as manic depression.

bipolar II disorder   a clinical condition in which episodes of major depression alternate with mildly manic periods. Typically the patient needs to be hospitalized during the depressed periods but not during the manic upswings.

bipolar III   a term used to describe a unipolar depressed person who develops mania or hypomania only with a psychopharmacologic challenge (i.e., after taking an antidepressant drug).

borderline personality disorder   a disorder characterized by a pattern of unstable and intense relationships, distorted self-image, difficulties with impulse control, and shifting extremes of emotion.

bulimia   an eating disorder characterized by eating binges followed by depression and self-criticism. In bulimia nervosa, eating binges are followed by vomiting and purging.

bupropion   the generic name for Wellbutrin.

Buspar   a nonhabit-forming antianxiety medication. Its generic name is buspirone.

buspirone   the generic name for Buspar.

butyrophenone   a family of antipsychotic medications such as Haldol.

carbamazepine   the generic name for Tegretol.

carbidopa   a substance that reduces the amount of levodopa (or l-dopa) required by patients suffering from Parkinsonism. Levodopa is converted into the neurotransmitter dopamine.

character those components of personality that are acquired.

chloral hydrate the generic name for a sleeping medication. Its trade name is Noctec.

chlorothiazide the generic name for Diuril.

Citalopram an SSRI antidepressant currently under development.

clinical depression a frequently used term for major depression.

clomipramine the generic name for Anafranil.

clonazepam the generic name for Klonopin.

clonidine an antihypertensive also used for narcotic withdrawal.

clorpromazine the generic name for Thorazine.

cogentin an anti-Parkinsonism medication. Its generic name is benztropine.

cognitive therapy a time-limited structured form of psychotherapy in which the goal is to change the negative, inaccurate ways the patient perceives the world, the self, and the future.

Coumadin an anticoagulant medication. Its generic name is warfarin.

cycloserine the generic name for the antibiotic Seromycin.

cyclothymia a form of manic depression characterized by relatively mild highs and lows.

Cytomel a thyroid hormone sometimes used to augment the effects of an antidepressant.

Dalmane a hypnotic agent or sleeping pill. It is a member of the benzodiazepine family of drugs. Its generic name is flurazepam.

Depakote an anticonvulsive medication and an alternative to lithium. Its generic name is valproic acid.

Deprenyl a European antidepressant. It is a monoamine oxidase inhibitor that lacks the cheese effect.

depression a bleak mood characterized by sadness, discouragement, hopelessness, despair. See major depression.

desipramine the generic name for Norpramin.

Desyrel an antidepressant structurally unlike the tricyclics, the monoamine oxidase inhibitors, and the selective serotonin re-uptake inhibitors. Its generic name is trazodone.

dexamethasone test a test in which a patient is given dexamethasone, after which the cortisol level is measured. Normally, dexamethasone suppresses the body's production of cortisol, but in some patients with major depression, the production of cortisol is unsuppressed and the serum cortisol rises.

diazepam the generic name for Valium.

digitoxin a cardiac medication extracted from *Digitalis purpurea*. Its chemical formula is $C_{41}H_{64}O_{13}$.

digoxin a cardiac medication extracted from the leaves of *Digitalis lanata*. Its chemical formula is $C_{41}H_{64}O_{14}$.

Diuril a diuretic and antihypertensive medication. Its generic name is chlorothiazide.

dopamine one of three major neurotransmitters found in the synapses of the brain. The other two are norepinephrine and serotonin.

double depression an episode of major depression that occurs on top of chronic, long-term mild depression.

DSM-IV an abbreviation for the fourth edition of the American Psychiatric Association's *Diagnostic and Statistical Manual of Mental Disorders*. The book lists symptoms for all psychiatric illnesses.

dysmorphic somatoform disorder obsessive concern with imaginary or exaggerated flaws in physical appearance.

dysphoria unpleasant mood associated with a shifting

set of symptoms including sadness, anxiety, and irritability.

dysthymia a mild but persistent form of depression, less severe in its symptoms than major depression but lasting at least two years (one year in children).

ECT the abbreviation for electroconvulsive therapy.

Effexor the trade name of venlafaxin.

EKG the abbreviation for electrocardiogram.

elation a strong, self-satisfied feeling of exhilaration, euphoria, and optimism.

Elavil a tricyclic antidepressant. Its generic name is amitriptyline.

FDA Food and Drug Administration.

fluoxetine the generic name of Prozac. The full generic name, fluoxetine hydrochloride, is also used.

fluvoxamine an SSRI antidepressant. Its trade name is Luvox.

formes frustes subclinical forms of a disorder characterized by one or a few symptoms rather than by the entire spectrum of symptoms.

generic drugs a drug not controlled by a manufacturer's trademark.

genetic equivalent a condition such as alcoholism, drug abuse, gambling, suicide, or sociopathy genetically linked to depression or manic depression.

grandiosity a delusional sense of superiority.

guanethidine an antihypertensive medication.

H_2-blockers medications that block histamine-2 receptors.

Halcion a short-acting hypnotic or sleeping pill of the benzodiazepine family. Its generic name is triazelam.

Haldol a butyrophenone antipsychotic medication also used to treat Tourette's Syndrome and hyperactivity in children. Its generic name is haloperidol.

half-life the time it takes for the amount of a drug in the blood to decrease by half.

hydralazine the generic name for Apresoline, an antihypertensive medication.

hyperthymia a mood characterized by high energy, confidence, and activity. Hyperthymia is a state that is more energetic than a normal good mood but less energetic or revved up than hypomania.

hypomania a mildly elevated, expansive mood lasting a few days. Hypomania is less intense than mania but more intense than hyperthymia.

hypothalamus a part of the brain responsible for regulation of autonomic activities including body temperature, sexual activity, hunger, and thirst.

hypothymia a mood in which the emotions and energy are slightly diminished.

imipramine the generic name for Tofranil.

interpersonal psychotherapy a time-limited structured form of psychotherapy designed to alleviate major depression.

IPT abbreviation for interpersonal psychotherapy.

isocarboxazid the generic name for Marplan.

kemadrine an anti-Parkinsonism medication.

Klonopin an antiseizure and antianxiety medication. It is a member of the benzodiazepine family of antianxiety medications. Its generic name is clonazepam.

L-trytophine an amino acid used to make serotonin.

levodopa the metabolic precursor of dopamine. Used in the treatment of Parkinson's disease.

levothyroxin thyroid hormone.

Librium an antianxiety agent and a member of the benzodiazepine family. Its generic name is chlordiazepoxide.

lithium an element which stabilizes the ups and downs of mood disorders by shifting the levels of water and electrolytes.

lorazepam the generic name for Ativan.

loxapine the generic name for Loxitane.

Loxitane   a tricyclic tranquilizer and antipsychotic drug.

Ludiomil   a tetracyclic antidepressant. Its generic name is maprotiline.

Luvox   an SSRI antidepressant. Its generic name is fluvoxamine.

major depression   an episode, at least two weeks in duration, characterized by many (not necessarily all) of the following symptoms: low feelings, loss of interest in life, inability to experience pleasure, difficulty concentrating, loss of energy, anxiety, changes in appetite and sleep patterns, and frequent thoughts about death and suicide. Also known as clinical depression or unipolar depression.

mania   a period of abnormal, persistent elation characterized by extreme talkativeness, rapid shifting from one idea to another, excitement, agitation, and hyperactivity.

manic depression   a disorder in which periods of moderate to severe depression alternate with unstable periods of elation. Also known as bipolar I disorder.

MAOI   abbreviation for monoamine oxidase inhibitors, a category of antidepressants.

maprotiline   the generic name for Ludiomil.

Marplan   a monoamine oxidase inhibitor antidepressant. Its generic name is isocarboxazid.

masked depression   a form of depression that is hidden behind physical symptoms for which no organic cause can be found.

Mellaril   an antipsychotic medication also used for the short-term treatment of depression with anxiety. Its generic name is thioridazine.

metabolite   the chemical compound produced by the breakdown of a drug in the body. The metabolite of Prozac is norfluoxetine.

methyldopa   the generic name for Aldomet, an antihypertensive drug.

Mianserin a tetracyclic antidepressant available in Europe.

Miltown a minor tranquilizer and antianxiety medication. It is no longer commonly used.

monoamine oxidase inhibitor a class of antidepressants that prevents the enzyme monoamine oxidase from degrading at the nerve endings in the brain. This in turn produces higher levels of norepinephrine and serotonin at the nerve synapses. Not to be taken with tyramine-containing foods such as cheese and Chianti wine.

mood the internal emotional outlook.

mood disorders a category of clinical conditions in which the patient feels a distressing lack of control over mood or emotions. Mood disorders affect the level of activity, cognitive abilities, patterns of sleep, appetite, sexuality, and, frequently, the patient's social and professional functioning.

moodswing an emotional state that fluctuates between the lows of depression and the highs of mania or hypomania.

Nardil a monoamine oxidase inhibitor antidepressant also used for panic disorders. Its generic name is phenelzine.

nefazadone the generic name for Serzone.

neurotransmitter a chemical substance that relays messages between nerves.

norepinephrine one of three major neurotransmitters found in the synapses of the brain. The other two are serotonin and dopamine.

norfluoxetine the metabolite of Prozac.

normal reactive depression relatively short-term depression connected to grief or bereavement.

Norpramin a tricyclic antidepressant. Its generic name is desipramine.

nortriptyline the generic name for the tricyclic antidepressants Pamelor and Aventyl.

obsessive compulsive disorder a clinical condition characterized by a distressing set of time-consuming repetitive thoughts and actions.

OCD abbreviation of obsessive compulsive disorder.

overdose an excessive or lethal amount of a drug.

Pamelor a tricyclic antidepressant. Its generic name is nortriptyline.

panic a severe attack of overwhelming anxiety.

Parnate a monoamine oxidase inhibitor antidepressant. Its generic name is tranylcypromine.

paroxetine the generic name for Paxil.

Paxil an SSRI antidepressant. Its generic name is paroxetine.

personality disorder a condition characterized by long-term inflexible and maladaptive patterns of distorted thought, perceptions, or behavior.

phenelzine the generic name for Nardil, an MAO inhibitor.

phenothiazine the generic name for a family of antipsychotic medications including Thorazine, Stelazine, and Mellaril.

phobia an anxiety disorder characterized by an irrational, persistent, exaggerated fear of a specific situation or object, combined with a compelling requirement to avoid the dreaded stimulus.

placebo a medication that is either completely or largely inert.

placebo effect the reactions of a patient to a medication that is inert. The physical and psychological consequences are thus created not by the drug itself but by the patient's expectations.

PMS abbreviation for premenstrual syndrome.

post-traumatic stress disorder a condition resulting from major trauma such as rape, childhood abuse, or wartime experiences, and including the reexperiencing of the trauma, emotional numbing, and other symptoms.

Prolixin a high-potency antipsychotic medication of the phenothiazine family. Its generic name is fluphenazine.

propranolol the generic name for Inderol, a beta-blocker antihypertensive also used for the treatment of heart tremors.

protriptyline the generic name for Vivactil.

Prozac an SSRI antidepressant. Its generic name is fluoxetine.

psychopharmacology the study of drugs that affect mental activity and emotional processes.

psychotropic drugs medications that affect the mood or mental processes.

PTSD abbreviation for post-traumatic stress disorder.

rapid cyclers manic depressives who experience four or more moodswings a year.

Raynaud's syndrome a medical syndrome in which the fingers turn color and become numb when exposed to cold.

REM abbreviation for rapid eye movement. Dreaming takes place during REM sleep.

reserpine an antihypertensive medication with anti-anxiety or tranquilizing properties.

Restoril a hypnotic or sleeping pill of the benzodiazepine family of antianxiety medications. Its generic name is temazepam.

Ritalin a psychostimulant often used for the treatment of attention deficit hyperactivity disorder. Its generic name is methylphenidate.

schizoaffective disorder a combination of major depression or mania with delusions or hallucinations.

secondary depression depression that occurs after or in response to a pre-existing medical or psychiatric disorder.

selective serotonin re-uptake inhibitors a class of antidepressants that operate by increasing the amount of serotonin in the synapses of the brain. Examples include Prozac, Paxil, and Zoloft.

Seromycin   an antibiotic medication. Its generic name is cycloserine.

Serzone   an SSRI antidepressant. Its generic name is nefazadone.

serotonin   one of three major neurotransmitters found in the synapses of the brain. The other two are norepinephrine and dopamine.

serotonin syndrome   an infrequent, potentially serious, systemic neurologic reaction to the combination of an SSRI antidepressant with another psychotropic drug.

sertraline   the generic name for Zoloft.

social phobia   fear of being scrutinized by others or of embarrassing oneself in public.

soft bipolar   a partial form of mania or hypomania with fewer symptoms than are required for the formal *DSM* diagnosis.

SSRI   abbrevation for selective serotonin re-uptake inhibitors.

Stelazine   a major anti-psychotic or tranquilizer of the phenothiazine family. Its generic name is trifluoperazine.

subclinical depression   a depressed condition in which the symptoms are not severe enough or numerous enough to merit a diagnosis of major depression or dysthymia.

Surmontil   a tricyclic antidepressant. Its generic name is trimipramine.

Survector   an antidepressant available in Europe. Its generic name is Amineptine.

Symmetrel   an anti-Parkinsonism medication also used for the prevention of influenza-A virus illness. Its generic name is amantadine.

synapse   the point where an impulse travels from one nerve to another: the gap between nerves.

T₃ triiodothyronine, a hormone produced by the thyroid gland. Sometimes given to augment an antidepressant.

TCA abbreviation for tricyclic antidepressants.

Tegretol an anticonvulsant drug. Its generic name is carbamazepine.

temazepam the generic name for Restoril.

temperament those aspects of personality that are innate or inherited.

Thorazine an antipsychotic of the phenothiazine family. Its generic name is clorpromazine.

Tofranil a tricyclic antidepressant. Its generic name is imipramine.

tolbutamide the generic name for Orinase, a medication used to lower blood glucose.

tranylcypromine the generic name for Parnate.

trazodone the generic name for Desyrel.

treatment-resistant depression depression that is unaffected by all major classes of antidepressants.

tricyclic antidepressants a class of antidepressants, so-called because the nucleus has a three-ring structure, that increases the level of norepinephrine and serotonin in the synapses of the brain.

triiodothyronine T₃, a thyroid hormone.

Trilafon an antipsychotic medication. Its generic name is perphenazine.

trimipramine the generic name for Surmontil.

unipolar depression a term for major depression. In contrast to bipolar disorder, unipolar depression is characterized by episodes of depression but not by periods of mania.

Valium an antianxiety medication and minor tranquilizer. Its generic name is diazepam.

valproic acid the generic name for Depakote, an anticonvulsive medication.

Venlafaxin a recently developed SSRI antidepressant. Its trade name is Effexor.

Vivactil   a tricyclic antidepressant. Its generic name is protriptyline.

warfarin   the generic name for Coumadin.

Wellbutrin   an antidepressant with a structure like that of the tricyclics, MAOIs, or SSRIs. Its generic name is bupropion.

withdrawal   the process of abstaining from a drug to which one has become habituated.

Xanax   an antianxiety medication and minor tranquilizer. Its generic name is alprazolam.

Zoloft   an SSRI antidepressant. Its generic name is sertraline.

• Appendix C •
Chapter References

Preface

Cohn, J.B.; Wilcox, C. A comparison of fluoxetine, imipramine, and placebo in patients with major depressive disorder. *J Clin Res* 46(3):26–31, 1985.

Stark, P.; Hardison, C.D. A review of multicenter controlled studies of fluoxetine versus imipramine and placebo in outpatients with major depressive disorder. *J Clin Psychiatry* 46(3):53–58, 1985.

Wernicke, J.F. The side effect profile and safety of fluoxetine. *J Clin Psychiatry* 46(3):59–67, 1985.

CHAPTER 1

Amit, Z.; Smith, B.R.; Gill, K. Serotonin uptake inhibitors: Effects on motivated consummatory behaviors. *J Clin Psychiatry* 52/12 (supp):55–60, 1991.

Bernstein, J.G. Induction of obesity by psychotropic drugs. *Ann N Y Acad Sci* 499:203–215, 1987.

Borys, D.J.; Setzer, S.C.; Ling, L.J.; Reisdorf, J.J; Day, L.C.; Krenzelok, E.P. Acute fluoxetine overdose: A report of 234 cases. *Am J Emerg Med* 10(2):115–20, 1992.

Boulas, C.; Kutcher, S.; Gardner, D.; Young, E. An open naturalistic trial of fluoxetine in adolescents and young adults with treatment-resistant major depression. *J Child Adolescent Psychopharmacol* 2/2:103-111, 1992.

Boyer, W.F. Potential indications for the selecive serotonin re-uptake inhibitors. *Int Clin Psychopharm* 6 (supp 5):5–12, 1992.

Cowley, Geoffrey, *et al.* "The Promise of Prozac," *Newsweek,* March 26, 1990.

Duke, Patty. *A Brilliant Madness: Living with Manic-Depressive Illness.* New York: Bantam Books, 1992.

Dunner, D.L. Diagnostic and treatment considerations in the depressed elderly patient. *Adv Ther* 9/6:350–359, 1992.

Feighner, J.P.; Boyer, W.F.; Meredith, C.H.; Hendrickson, G. An overview of fluoxetine in geriatric depression. *Br J Psychiatry* 153 (supp 3):105–108, 1988.

Ferreira, L.; Soares Da Silva, P. 5-Hydroxytryptamine and alcoholism. *Hum Psychopharmacol* 6/supp: S21–S24, 1991.

Fieve, R.R.; Rosenthal, D.; Brill, H., eds. *Genetics and Research in Psychiatry,* Baltimore: Johns Hopkins University Press, 1975.

Fuller, R.W.; Schaffer, R.J.; Roush, B.W.; Molloy, B.B. Drug disposition as a factor in the lowering of brain serotonin by chloroamphetamines in the rat. *Biochem Pharmacol* 21:1413–1417, 1972.

Gordon, George and Bradberry, Grace. "Is this pill a miracle or a mind bender?" *Daily Mail,* October 27, 1990.

Hellerstein, D.J.; Yanowitch, P.; Rosenthal, J.; Samstag, L.W.; Maurer, M.; Kasch, K.; Burrows, L.; Poster, M.; Cantillon, M; Winston, A. A randomized double-blind study of fluoxetine versus placebo in the treatment of dysthymia. *Am J Psychiatry* 150(8): 1169–1975, 1993.

Holden, C. Depression: The News Isn't Depressing. *Science* 254; 1450–1452, 1991.

Kramer, Peter C. *Listening to Prozac.* New York: Viking, 1993.

Kuhn, R. The treament of depressive states with G22355 (imipramine hydrochloride). *Am J Psychiatry.* 115:459–464, 1958.

Kupfer, D.J. Long-term treatment of depression. *J Clin Psychiatry* 52/5(supp):28–34.

Markowitz, P.J. Drug treatment of personality disorders. *Br J Psychiatry* 162:122–131, 1993.

Miller, Michael W. "A New Antidepressant Will Challenge Prozac." *The Wall Street Journal,* December 29, 1993.

Montgomery, S.A., *et al.* A double-blind, placebo-controlled study of fluoxetine in patients with DSM-III-R obsessive-compulsive disorder. *Eur Neuropsychopharmacol* 3(2): 143–52, 1993.

Montgomery, S.A.; Dufour, H.; Brion, S.; *et al.* The prophylactic efficacy of fluoxetine in unipolar depression. *Br J Psychiatry* 153(supp 3):69–76, 1988.

Nordon, M.J. Fluoxetine in borderline personality disorder. *Progress in Neuro-Psychopharm and Biol Psychiatry* 13:885–893, 1989.

Pigott, T.A.; Pato, M.T.; Bernstein, S.E.; Grover, G.N.; Hill, L.J.; Tolliver, T.J.; Murphy, D.L. Controlled comparisons of clomipramine and fluoxetine in the treatment of obsessive-compulsive disorder: Behavioral and biological results. *Arch Gen Psychiatry* 47:926–932, 1990.

Pollack, M.H.; Rosenbaum, J.F. Fluoxetine treatment of cocaine abuse in heroin addicts. *J Clin Psychiatry* 52/1:31–33, 1991.

Rimer, S. With millions taking Prozac, a legal culture arises. *The New York Times,* December 13, 1993.

Simeon, J.D.; Dinicola, V.E.; Ferguson, B.H.; Copping, W. Adolescent depression: A placebo-controlled fluoxetine treatment study and follow-up. *Prog in Neuropsychopharmacol Biol Psychiatry* 14(5): 791–795.

Simpson, S.G.; DePaulo, J.R. Fluoxetine treatment of bipolar II depression. *J Clin Psychopharmacol* 11/1:52–54, 1991.

Stark, R.; Hardison, C.D. A review of multicenter controlled studies of fluoxetine versus imipramine and placebo in outpatients with major depressive disorder. *J Clin Psychiatry* 46(3):53–58, 1985.

Stokes, P.E. Fluoxetine: A five-year review. *Clin Ther* 15/2:216–243, 1993.

Styron, William. *Darkness Visible: A Memoir of Madness.* New York: Random House, 1990.

Toufexis, Anastasia. "The Personality Pill." *Time,* October 11, 1993.

Venkataraman, S.; Naylor, M.W.; King, C.A. Mania associated with fluoxetine treatment in adolescents. *J Am Acad Child Adolesc Psychiatry* 31/2:276–281, 1992.

Walsh, B.T. Fluoxetine treatment of bulimia nervosa. *J Psychosomatic Res* 35(supp 1):33–40, 1991.

Wong, D.T.; Horn, J.S.; Fuller, R.W. Kinetics of serotonin accumulation into synaptosomes of rat brain—effects of amphetamines and chloroamphetamines. *Biochem Pharmacol* 22:311–322, 1973.

CHAPTER 2

Akiskal, H.S.; Akiskal, K. Cyclothymic, hyperthymic and depressive temperaments as subaffective variants of mood disorders. In: Tasman, A.; Riba, M.B.,

(Eds.) *American Psychiatric Press Review of Psychiatry* 11: 43–62, 1992.

Akiskal, H.S. [The depressive before depression] La deprime avant la depression. *L'Encephale* 18/4(spec): 485–489, 1992.

Akiskal, H.S. New insight into the nature and heterogeneity of mood disorders. *J Clin Psychiatry* 50/May(supp):6–10; discussion 11–2, 1990.

Akiskal, H.S. The clinical spectrum of so-called "minor" depressions. *Am J Psychotherapy* 46/1:9–22, 1992.

Akiskal, H.S. The distinctive mixed states of bipolar I, II, III. *Clin Neuropharmacol* 15/1(supp, Pt. A): 632A–633A.

Bittman, B.J.; Young, R.C. Mania in elderly man treated with bupropion [letter]. *Am J Psychiatry* 148/4:541, 1991.

Boyer, W.F. Potential indications for the selective serotonin re-uptake inhibitors. *Int Clin Psychopharmacol* 6/5(supp):5–12, 1992.

Costello, C.G.; Scott, C.B. Primary and secondary depression: A review. *Can J Psychiatry* 36/3:210–217, 1991.

DSM-IV Draft Criteria: Task Force on DSM-IV. Washington, D.C., American Psychiatric Press, 1993.

Dunner, D.L.; Patrick, V.; Fieve, R.R. Rapid cycling manic depressive patients. *Compr Psychiatry,* 18: 562–566, 1977.

Feder, R. Fluoxetine-induced mania. *J Clin Psychiatry* 51/12:524–525, 1990.

Feighner, J.P. A Comparative Trial of Fluoxetine and Amitriptyline in Patients with Major Depressive Disorder. *J Clin Psychiatry* 46:369–372, 1985.

Fieve, R. *Moodswing*. New York: William Morrow, 1989.

Fieve, R. *Physician's Guide to Depression*. New York: PW Communications, Inc., 1975.

Fieve, R. and Dunner. *Unipolar and Bipolar Affective States in the Nature and Treatment of Depression.* New York: John Wiley, 1975.

Fluoxetine Bulimia Nervosa Collaborative Study Group. Fluoxetine in the treatment of bulimia nervosa. *Arch Gen Psychiatry* 49:139–147, 1992.

Goodman, F.K.; Jamison, K.R. *Manic Depressive Illness.* New York: Oxford University Press, 1990.

Greist, J.H.; Jefferson, J.W. *Depression and Its Treatment.* Revised edition. Washington, D.C.: American Psychiatric Press, Inc., 1992.

Hadley, A.; Cason, M.P. Mania resulting from lithium-fluoxetine combination [letter]. *Am J Psychiatry* 146:1637–1638, 1989.

Jerome, L. Hypomania with fluoxetine. *J Am Acad Child Adolesc Psychiatry* 30/5:850–851, 1991.

Joffe, R.T.; Levitt, A.J.; Bagby, R.M.; Regan, J.J. Clinical features of situational and nonsituational major depression. *Psychopathology* 26/3–4:138–144, 1993.

Kaplan, Harold I., and Sadock, Benjamin J. *Synopsis of Psychiatry,* 6th ed. Baltimore: Williams and Wilkins, 1991.

Keller, M.B.; Lavori, P.W.; Endicott, J.; Coryell, W.; Klerman, G.L. "Double depression": Two-year follow-up. *Am J Psychiatry* 140:98–100, 1986.

Klein, D.F.; Wender, P.H. *Understanding Depression: A Complete Guide to its Diagnosis and Treatment.* New York: Oxford University Press, 1993.

Klein, D.N.; Taylor, E.B.; Harding, K.; *et al.* Double depression and episodic major depression: demographic, clinical, familial, personality, and socioenvironmental characteristics and short-term outcome. *Am J Psychiatry* 145:1226–1231, 1988.

Klerman, G.L.; Weisman, M.M. Increasing rates of depression. *JAMA* 261:2229–2235, 1989.

Lebegue, B. Mania precipitated by fluoxetine [letter]. *Am J Psychiatry* 144:1620, 1987.

Liebowitz, M.R.; Quitkin, F.M.; Stewart, J.W.; *et al.* Antidepressant specificity in atypical depression. *Arch Gen Psychiatry* 45:129–137.

Moras, K.; Barlow, D. Secondary Depression: Definition and treatment. *Psychopharm Bull* 28/1:27–33, 1992.

Nierenberg, A.A.; Amsterdam, J.D. Treatment-resistant depression: Definition and treatment approaches. *J Clin Psychiatry* 51/6(supp):39–50(discussion), 1990.

Piredda, S.G.; Rubinstein, S.L. Hypomania induced by fluoxetine. *Biol Psychiatry* 32/1:107, 1992.

Post, R.M. Non-lithium treatment for bipolar disorder. *J Clin Psychiatry* 51/8 (supp):9–16, 1990.

Potter, W.Z.; Ketter, T.A. Pharmacological issues in the treatment of bipolar disorder: Focus on mood-stabilizing compounds. *Can J Psychiatry* 38/2(supp): 51–56, 1993.

Quitkin, F.M.; McGrath, P.J.; Stewart, J.W.; Harrison, W.; Wager, S.G.; Nunes, E.; Rabkin, J.G.; Tricamo, E.; Markowitz, J.; Klein, D.F. Phenelzine and imipramine in mood reactive depressives. Further delineation of the syndrome of atypical depression. *Arch Gen Psychiatry* 46/9:787–93, 1989.

Reynolds, C.F. Treatment of depression in special populations. *J Clin Psychiatry* 53/9:45–53, 1992.

Schneier, F.R; Liebowitz, M.R.; Davies, S.O.; Fairbanks, J.; Hollander, E.; Campeas, R.; Klein, D.F. Fluoxetine in panic disorder. *J Clin Psychopharmacol* 10/2:119–121, 1990.

Spitzer, R.L.; Endicott, J.; Robins, E. Research Diagnostic Criteria: Rationale and reliability. *Arch Gen Psychiatry* 35:773–782, 1978.

Stokes, P.E. Fluoxetine: A five-year review. *Clin Ther* 15/2:216–243, 1993.

Wehr, T.A.; Goodwin, F.K. Can antidepressants cause

mania and worsen the course of affective illness? *Am J Psychiatry* 144/11:1403–1411, 1987.

Weisler, R.H. Treatment strategies for lithium-resistant bipolar depression. *J Clin Psychiatry Monograph* 10/1:27–36, 1990.

Winokur, G. The concept of secondary depression and its relationship to comorbidity. *Psychiatry Clin North Am* 13/4:567–583, 1990.

Wise, M.G.; Taylor, S.E. Anxiety and mood disorders in medically ill patients. *J Clin Psychiatry* 51/1: 27–32, 1990.

Zisook, S. Treatment of Dysthymia and Atypical Depression. *J Clin Psychiatry* 10/1:15–26.

Zubieta, J.K.; Demitrack, M.A. Possible bupropion precipitation of mania and a mixed affective state [letter]. *J Clin Psychopharmacol* 11/5:327–328.

CHAPTER 3

Altamura, A.C.; Montgomery, S.A.; Wernicke, J.F. The evidence for 20-mg a day of fluoxetine as the optimal dose in the treatment of depression. *Br J Psychiatry* 153/3(supp):109–112, 1988.

Benfield, P.; Heel, R.C.; Lewis, S.P. Fluoxetine: A review of its pharmacodynamic and pharmacokinetic properties, and therapeutic efficacy in depressive illness. *Drug* 32:481–508, 1986.

Bunney, W.E.; Davis, J. Norepinephrine in depressive reactions. *Arch Gen Psychiatry* 13:483–494, 1965.

Cooper, G.L. The safety of fluoxetine—an update. *Br J Psychiatry* 153/3(supp):77–86, 1988.

Henry, J.A. Toxicity of antidepressants: Comparison with fluoxetine. *Int Clin Psychopharma* 6/6(supp): 22–27, 1992.

Kupfer, D.J. Long-term treatment of depression. *J Clin Psychiatry* 52/5(supp):28–34.

Naranjo, Claudio, *et al.* Fluoxetine differentially alters

alcohol intake and other consummatory behaviors in problem drinkers. *Clin Pharmacol Ther*, April, 1990.

Preskorn, S.H.; Burke, M. Somatic therapy for major depressive disorder: Selection of an antidepressant. *J Clin Psychiatry* 53/9(supp):5–18, 1992.

Richelson, Elliot, M.D. *Antidepressants and Receptor Theory: Concepts and Reality.* Dista Products Company, 1990.

Rudorfer, M.V.; Potter, W.Z. Antidepressants. A comparative review of the clinical pharmacology and therapeutic use of the "newer" versus the "older" drugs. *Drugs* 37/5:713–38, 1989.

Schatberg, A.F. Dosing stategies for antidepressant agents. *J Clin Psychiatry* 52/5(supp):14–20, 1991.

Schildkraut, J. The catecholamine hypothesis of affective disorder: A review of supporting evidence. *Am J Psychiatry* 122:509–522, 1965.

Stark, P.; Fuller, R.W.; Wong, D.T. The pharmacologic profile of fluoxetine. *J Clin Psychiatry* 46:7–13, 1985.

Stark, P.; Hardison, C.D. A review of multicenter controlled studies of fluoxetine versus imipramine and placebo in outpatients with major depressive disorder. *J Clin Psychiatry* 46(3):53–58, 1985.

Stokes, P. The changing horizon in the treatment of depression: Scientific/clinical publication overview. *J Clin Psychiatry* 52/5(supp):35–43, 1991.

Wernicke, J.F.; Bremner, J.D. Fluoxetine effective in the long-term treatment of depression. *Br J Clin Pract* 40/46(supp):17–23, 1986.

CHAPTER 4

Balon, Richard; Yeragani, Vikram K.; Pohl, Robert; and Ramesh, C. Sexual Dysfunction During Antidepressant Treatment. *J Clin Psychiatry* 54:67, June 1993.

Cooper, Glenn L. The safety of fluoxetine—an update. *Br J Psychiatry* 153/3(supp):77–86, 1988.

Dursum, S.; *et al.* Toxic serotonin symptom after fluoxetine plus carbamazepine [letter]. *Lancet* 342 (August 14):442–443, 1993.

Fawcett, Jan. M.D., *et al. A Rational Approach to Antidepressant Drug Selection,* Eli Lilly and Company, 1993.

Fluoxetine Bulimia Nervosa Collaborative Study Group. Fluoxetine in the Treatment of Bulimia nervosa. *Arch Gen Psychiatry,* Vol. 49, February 1992.

Hollander, Eric, M.D., and McCarley, Allison. Yohimbine Treatment of Sexual Side Effects Induced by Serotonin Reuptake Blockers. *J Clin Psychiatry* 53:207–209, 1992.

Musher, J.S. Anorgasmia with the use of fluoxetine [letter]. *Am J Psychiatry* 147:948, 1990.

Pearson, H. Interaction of fluoxetine with carbazepine [letter]. *J Clin Psychiatry* 51:126, 1990.

Prozac Comprehensive Monograph. Dista Products Company, Eli Lilly and Co. April 1993.

Richelson, Elliot, M.D. *Antidepressants and Receptor Theory,* Dista Products Co., Eli Lilly and Company.

Smith, D.; Levitte, S. Assocation of fluozetine and return of sexual potency in three elderly men. *J Clin Psychiatry* 54 (August):317–319, 1993. From the Portland Veterans Administration Medical Center, Portland, Oregon.

Stokes, P.E. Fluoxetine: A five-year review. *Clin Ther* 15/2:216–243, 1993.

Zajecka, John; Fawcett, Jan; Schaff, Mary; Jeffriess, Helen; and Guy, Charles. The Role of Serotonin in Sexual Dysfunction: Fluoxetine-Associated Orgasm Dysfunction. *J Clin Psychiatry* 52:2, 66–68, February 1991.

CHAPTER 5

Bergstrom, R.F.; Lemberger, L.; Farid, N.A.; Wolen, R.L. Clinical pharmacology and pharmacokinetics of fluoxetine: A Review. *Br J Psychiatry* 153(supp 3):47–50, 1988.

Fisch, C. Effect of fluoxetine on the electro-cardiogram. *J Clin Psychiatry* 46 (no. 3, sec 2):42–44, 1985.

Goodnick, Paul J., M.D. and Nancy G. Klimas, M.D. *Chronic Fatigue and Related Immuno Syndromes*, Washington, D.C.: American Psychiatric Press, 1993.

Schou, M.; Weinstein, M.R. Problems of lithium maintenance during pregancy, delivery, and lactation. *Agressologie* 21, A:7–9, 1980.

CHAPTER 6

Beasley, *et al.*, *British Medical Journal* 303 (September 21):685–692, 1991.

Burton, Thomas M. Medical Flap: Anti-Depression Drug of Eli Lilly Loses Sales After Attack by Sect, *Wall Street Journal*, April 19, 1991.

Burton, Thomas M. Scientologists Fail to Persuade FDA on Prozac. *Wall Street Journal,* August 2, 1991.

Fava, Maurizio, M.D., and Rosenbaum, Jerrold F., M.D. Suicidality and Fluoxetine: Is There a Relationship? *Journal of Clinical Psychiatry,* Vol. 52, No. 3, pp. 108–111, p. 108, March 1991.

Fava, Maurizio, M.D.; Rosenbaum, Jerrold F., M.D.; Pava, Joel A., Ph.D.; McCarthy, Mary K., M.D.; Ronald J. Steingard, M.D., and Bouffides, Evan, M.A. Anger Attacks in Unipolar Depression, Part I: Clinical Correlates and Response to Fluoxetine Treament. *Am J Psychiatry* 150:8, pp. 1158–1163, August 1993.

Freudenheim, Milt. The Drug Makers Are Listening to Prozac. *The New York Times*, January 9, 1993.

Funk and Wagnall's New Comprehensive International Dictionary. Newark, New Jersey: International Press, 1984.

Goodwin, Frederick K. and Jamison, Kay Redfield. *Manic-Depressive Illness*. New York: Oxford University Press, 1990.

Kaplan, Harold I. and Sadock, Benjamin J. *Synopsis of Psychiatry*, 6th ed. Baltimore: Williams and Wilkins, 1991.

Karel, Richard. Members React to Campaign Discrediting Prozac, Psychiatry. *Psychiatric News*, Col XXVI, No. 11, June 7, 1991.

Murphy, Todd. Louisville Woman's Suit Over Prozac is Dismissed. *The Courier-Journal*, October 1, 1992.

Papolos, Demitri, M.D., and Papolos, Janice. *Overcoming Depression*, Revised Edition. New York: HarperPerennial, 1992.

Prozac: The Building of a Smear Campaign. *The Illinois Pharmacist*, July 1991.

Sherman, Brian. A Mindless Attack on Modern Medicine. *Private Practice*, October 1991.

Styron, William, *Darkness Visible: A Memoir of Madness*. New York: Random House, 1990.

CHAPTER 7

Baldessarini, R.J. Current status of antidepressants: clinical pharmacology and therapy. *J Clin Psychiatry*, 1989; 50: 117–126. *In Depression: The Economic Impact*, Dista Products Co., 1992.

Berken, G.H.; Weinstein, D.O.; Stern, W.C. Weight Gain: a side effect of tricyclic antidepressants. *J Affective Disord* 1984; 7:133–138, in *J Clin Psychiatry* Monograph 1–:1 May 1992.

Burke, Karen E., M.D., Ph.D. Health Up-Date: Depression: New Antidepressant Treatment Options, *Diplomatic World Bulliten,* April 19–26, 1993.

Cooper, Glenn L. The Safety of Fluoxetine—An Update, *British Journal of Psychiatry* 153 (suppl. 3): 77–86, 1988.

Greist, John H., M.D., and Jefferson, James W., M.D. *Depression and Its Treatment.* Prozac Comprehensive Monograph, 1993.

Rush, A. John, M.D. Problems Associated with Diagnosis of Depression. *J Clin Psychiatry* 1990; 51 (6, supp):15–22.

Sackett, D.L.; Haynes, R.B.; Tugwell, P., eds. *Clinical Epidemiology: A Basic Science for Clinical Medicine.* Boston: Little, Brown, 1985.

Shapiro, S.; Skinner, E.A.; Kesslper, E.A.; *et al.* Utilization of health and mental health services: Three Epidemiologic Catchment Area Sites. *Arch Gen Psychiatry* 41:971–978, 1984.

Sternbach, H. The serotonin syndrome. *Am J Psychiatry* 148:705–713, 1991.

Styron, William. *Darkness Visible.* New York: Random House, 1990.

Wells, K.B.; Stewart, A.; Hays, R.D.; *et al.* The functioning and well-being of depressed patients: Results from the Medical Outcomes study. *JAMA* 262: 914–919, 1989.

Wells, K.B.; Hays, R.D.; Burnam, M.A.; *et al.* Detection of depressive disorder for patients receiving prepaid or fee-for-service care: Results from the Medical Outcomes Study. *JAMA* 262:3298-3302, 1981.

Zung, W.W.K. The role of rating scales in the identification and management of the depressed patient in the primary care setting. *J Clin Psychiatry* 51 (supp 6):72–76, 1991.

CHAPTER 8

Akiskal, H.S. "The Distinctive Mixed States of Bipolar I, II, III." *Clin Neuropharm* 15 supp 1:632A–633A, 1992.

Akiskal, H.S., M.D. Depression in Cyclothymic and Related Temperaments, Clinical and Pharmacologic Considerations. *J Clin Psychiatry*. Monograph 10:1, May 1992.

Akiskal, Hagop S. M.D. Depression in Cyclothymic and Related Temperaments. Clinical and Pharmacologic Considerations. *J Clin Psychiatry*. Monograph 10:1, May 1992.

Akiskal, Hagop S., M.D.; Adib H. Bitar, M.D.; Vahe R. Puzantian, M.D.; Ted L. Rosenthal, Ph.D.; Parks W. Walker, M.D. The Nosological Status of Neurotic Depression. *Arch General Psychiatry,* 35:756–766, 1978.

Akiskal, Hagop S.; Cassano, G.B.; Musetti, L.; Perugi, G.; Tundo, A.; Mignani, V. Psychopathology, temperament, and past course in primary major depressions 1. Review of evidence for a bipolar spectrum. *Psychopathology* 22/5:268–77, 1989.

Andreasen, N.C. Creativity and mental illness: Prevalence rates in writers and their first-degree relatives. *Am J Psychiatry* 144:1288–1292, 1987.

Angier, Natalie. An Old Idea About Genius Wins New Scientific Support. *New York Times,* October 12, 1993.

Cloninger, C.P. "A General Model of Personality and Psychopathology Speech." *Presidential Address at 1993 American Psychological Association.*

Dunner, D.L.; Patrick, V.; Fieve, R.R. Rapic cycling manic depressive patients. *Compr Psychiatry* 18: 561–566, 1977.

Fieve, Ronald R. *Moodswing.* New York: William Morrow, 1989.

Fieve, R.; Rosenthal, D. and Brill, H. *Genetic Research and Psychiatry.* Johns Hopkins University Press, 1978.

Fieve, Ronald R. "Search for Biological/Genetic Markers in a Long-term Epidemiological and Morbid Risk Study of Effective Disorder." *Journal of Psychiatric Research* 18, no. 4, 1984.

Goodwin, Frederick K. and Kay Redfield Jamison. *Manic-Depressive Illness.* New York: Oxford University Press, 1990.

Hollander, E.; Leibowitz, M.R.; Winchel, R.; Klumker, A.; Klein, D.F. Treatment of body dysmorphic disorder with serotonin re-uptake blockers. *Am J Psychiatry* 146:768, 1989.

Jamison, K.R. *Touch of Fire.* 1993.

Kaplan, Harold I. and Sadock, Benjamin J. *Synopsis of Psychiatry,* 6th ed. Baltimore: Williams and Wilkins, 1991.

Kendler, K.S.; Neale, M.C.; Kessler, R.C; Heath, A.C.; Phil, D.; Eaves, L.J. "Major depression and generalized anxiety disorder: Same genes (partly) different environments?" *Arch Gen Psychiatry,* 49:716–722, 1992.

Kendler, K.S. "Risk Factors in the Familial Aggregation of Psychiatric Disorders." *Psychosomatic Medicine* 20 (no. 2): 311–319, 1990.

Kidd, J.R.; Kidd, K.K.; Weiss, K.M. "Human Genome Diversity Initiative." *Human Biology* 65(1): 1–6., February 1993.

Klein, Donald F. and Paul H. Wender. *Understanding Depression: Complete Guide to Its Diagnosis and Treatment.* Oxford University Press, 1993.

Mendlewicz, J.; Papadimitriou, G.; Wilmotte, J. "Family Study of Panic Disorder: Comparison with Generalized Anxiety Disorder, Major Depression, and Normal Subjects." *Psychiatr Genet* 3/2:73–78, 1993.

Mendlewicz, J., S. Sevy, K. Mendelbaum, "Minireview:

Molecular Genetics in Affective Illness." *Life Sci* 52/3:231–42, 1993.

Oldham, J.M. and L.B. Morris. *The Patient: A Self-Portrait: Why You Think, Love, and Act the Way You Do.* New York: Bantam Books, 1990.

Politin, P.; Fieve, R.R. Patient rejection of lithium carbonate prophylaxis. *JAMA* 218:864–866, 1971.

Salzman, Carl, M.D. The Current Status of Fluoxetine. *Neuropsychopharmacology,* vol. 7, no. 4, 1992.

Stone, Michael H. *Abnormalities of Personality.* New York: W.W. Norton and Company, 1993.

Winokur, G.; Coryell, W.; Endicott, J.; Akiskal, H. "Further Distinctions Between Manic-Depressive Illness (Bipolar Disorder) and Primary Depressive Disorder (Unipolar Depression)." *American Journal of Psychiatry* 150 (8):1176–81, August 1993.

Winokur, G.; Clayton, P.; Reich, T. *Manic-Depressive Illness.* New York; Mosby, 1969.

CHAPTER 9

Akiskal, H.S; Walker, P.; Puzantian, V.; King, D.; Rosenthal, T.L.; Dranon, M. "Bipolar Outcome in the Course of Depressive Illness." *J Affect Dis* 5:115–128, 1983.

Boulos, Carolyn, M.D.; Stan Kutcher, M.D.; David Gardner, B. Sc.; Ellen Young, R.N. An Open Naturalistic Trial of Fluoxetine in Adolescents and Young Adults with Treatment-Resistant Major Depression. *Journal of Child & Adolescent Psychopharmacology,* vol 2. no. 2: 103–11, 1992.

Fawcett, Jan, M.D.; Jerrold F. Rosenbaum, M.D.; Alan F. Schatzberg, M.D.; and John M. Zajecka, M.D. Consultations in Clinical Psychopharmacology: A Rational Approach to Antidepressant Drug Selection, Eli Lilly August 1993.

Feighner, J.P., *et al.* An Overview of Fluoxetine in

Geriatric Depression. *British Journal of Psychiatry* 153 (supp. 3):105–108, 1988

Jenike, M.A.; Baer, C.; Greist, J.H. Clomipramine versus fluoxetine in obsessive-compulsive disorder: A retrospective comparison of side effects and efficacy. *J Clin Psychopharmacol* 10:122–124, 1990.

Kaplan, Harold I. and Sadock, Benjamin J. *Synopsis of Psychiatry*, 6th ed. Baltimore: Williams and Wilkins, 1991.

Kupfer, David J., M.D. Long-term Treatment of Depression. *J Clin Psychiatry* vol 52, no. 5 (supp.):28–34 May 1991.

Prien, R.F.; Kupfer, D.J. Continuation drug therapy for major depressive episodes: how long should it be maintained? *Am J Psychiatry* 143:18–23, 1986.

Scheier, F.R; Liebowitz, M.R.; Davies, S.O.; Fairbanks, *et al.* Fluoxetine in panic disorder. *J Clin Psychopharmacol* 10:119–121, 1990.

Upward, J.W.; Edwards, J.G.; Goldie, Ann; Waller, D.G. Comparative Effects of Fluoxetine and Amitriptyline on Cardiac Function. *Br J Clin Pharmacol* 26:399–402, 1988.

Venkataraman, Sanjeev; Michael W. Naylor and Cheryl A. King. Mania Associated with Fluoxetine Treatment in Adolescents. *J Am Acad Child Adolesc Psychiatry* 31:2 276–281, March 1992.

CHAPTER 10

Akiskal, H.S.; Cassano, G.B.; Musetti, L.; Perugi, G.; Tundo, A.; Mignani, V. Psychopathology, temperament, and past course in primary major depressions 1. Review of evidence for a bipolar spectrum. *Psychopathology* 22/5:268–77, 1989.

Akiskal, H.S. The distinctive mixed states of Bipolar I, II, III. *Clin Neuropharm* 15/Supp 1:632A–633A, 1992.

Ballus, C.; Gaston, C. Evaluation clinique des nouveaux anti-dépresseurs. *L'encephale* vol 7, no. 1. 133–137, May-June 1991.

Fieve, R.R.; Goodnick, P.J; Peselow, E.D.; Barouche, F.; Schlegel, A. "Pattern Analysis of Antidepressant Response to Fluoxetine." *J Clin Psychiatry* 47/11:560–562, 1986.

Fieve, R.R.; Goodnick, P.J.; Peselow, E.D.; Schlegel, A. Fluoxetine response: Endpoint versus pattern analysis. *Int Clin Psychopharm* 1:320–323, 1986.

Freudenheim, Milt. The Drug Makers Are Listening to Prozac. *The New York Times,* January 9, 1993.

Miller, Michael W. "A New Antidepressant Will Challenge Prozac." *The Wall Street Journal,* December 29, 1993.

Snyder, Solomon H. *The New Biology of Mood.* New York: Pfizer, 1988.

Index